Eggs in your life

Feed-Food Ltd
53 Dongola Road, Ayr,
KA7 3BN, Scotland, UK

First published 2013
Printed 2013

British Library Cataloguing in Publication Data
Eggs in your life

ISBN: 978-0-9575496-0-9

Disclaimer
Every reasonable effort has been made to ensure that the material in this
book is true, correct, complete and appropriate at the time of writing.
Nevertheless the publishers, the editors, and the authors do not accept
responsibility for any omission or error, or for any injury, damage, loss or
financial consequences arising from the use of the book.

Typeset by Feed-Food Ltd, Ayr
Cover image: http://www.flickr.com/photos/wiredwitch/4495285806/

EGGS IN YOUR LIFE

Peter Surai and Ray Noble

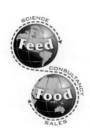 **Feed-Food Ltd**

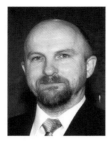

Dr. Peter Surai started his studies at Kharkov University, Ukraine, where he obtained his PhD and DSc in biochemistry studying effects of antioxidants on poultry. Later he became Professor of Human Physiology. In 1994 he moved to Scotland to continue his antioxidant related research in poultry and in 2000 he was promoted to a full Professor of Nutritional Biochemistry at the Scottish Agricultural College. Now he is a visiting professor there. Recently he was awarded Honorary Professorships in 5 universities in various countries. In 2010 he was elected to the Russian Academy of Agricultural Science as a foreign member. He has more than 650 research publications, including 125 papers in peer-reviewed journals and 8 books. In 1999 he received the prestigious John Logie Baird Award for Innovation for the development of "super-eggs" and, in 2000, The World's Poultry Science Association Award for Research in recognition of an outstanding contribution to the development of the poultry industry. For the last 10 years he has been lecturing all over the world visiting 70 countries.

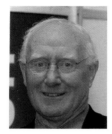

Ray Noble holds an Honours Degree in Agricultural Biochemistry from the University of Durham and a Ph.D. for his study on the effects of gonadal hormones on aspects of avian mineral metabolism using radioisotopes. He was awarded a D.Sc. by the University of Newcastle for research and published work on lipid metabolism. His career has covered basic biochemical research with additional teaching involvements at graduate and postgraduate levels. In 1989 he was appointed to be Head and Professor of the Department of Biochemical Sciences at the Scottish Agricultural College. His major areas of interest embrace lipid metabolism in mammalian and avian species, male infertility and sperm function, nutrition and health and radiotracer methodology. He is author of more than 440 original research papers, chapters and reviews and has been the recipient of a wide range of national and international awards, research funding, sponsorships and consultancies. He is involved in fifteen national/international patents in various aspects of biotechnology. His personal awards include an International Atomic Energy Award, a Scottish Institute of Bankers Prize, the Tom Newman Memorial Medal and International Award for meritorious contribution to avian research and Scottish Food and Drink Award for Best New Innovative Product.

CONTENTS

An egg a day
keeps diseases at bay

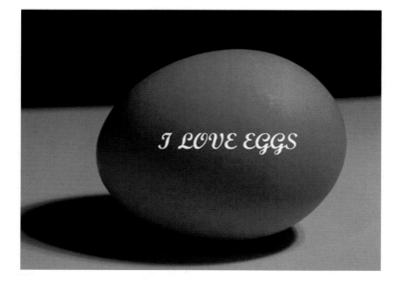

The egg is "an axisymmetric elliptical spheroid reproductive body produced by females of animals, enclosed in a protective layer and capable of developing into a new individual"

Oxford English Dictionary

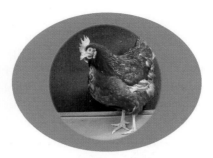

PREFACE

Which came first, the chicken or the egg? Answer - the egg of course. The egg existed some hundreds of millions years before the chicken as a format for the reproduction of the first land-dwelling animals - the reptiles. The present day chicken's egg is a highly refined version of this reproductive adaptation to life on land, making its appearance a mere four or five thousand years ago. The subsequent period has been more than enough for the egg to be seen as possessing a unique range of properties from which we can take full advantage. These include:

- ceremonial rituals and traditions, symbolic and otherwise - many of which, after centuries, still remain as vital and significant components of present day annual celebrations and ceremonies, for example the commemoration of religious and social events (Easter, births, marriages etc).

- a source of compounds and chemicals to satisfy specific aspects of manufacturing and commercial interests, for example polymers, pharmaceuticals etc.

But most significant is their extensive role in our past and present diet

Although it was never the intention that the egg be eaten, eggs have been a staple component of the human diet since the earliest of times. From the hunter-gatherers collecting wild bird eggs, to the domestication of the jungle fowl, which ultimately led to the present-day bird, able to deliver a stable, reliable and consistently high supply of eggs. The roles of the egg within the modern diet are such that it has to be considered to date as one of the most versatile ingredients in our nutrition.

The egg is still referred to as "humble" but its value and input to our general and specific dietary requirements are such that the term is quite inappropriate. With worldwide annual egg production now exceeding some sixty million metric tons from a total laying flock of approximately six and a half billion hens, the role of the contemporary laying bird has come a very long way from its origins.

However, under the eagle eye of contemporary nutritional science and interpretative abilities, the egg has most recently been at the receiving end of highly vocal criticism. This is in spite of the nutritional acceptability of the egg having been the subject of the most rigorous statistical test that could ever be devised in terms of time (thousands of years) and replication (a world based population). Surely this is proof enough for an unblemished nutritional role for the egg - or has there existed a fault line all along? As an interested reader and consumer, you are invited to read on. . .

Peter Surai and Ray Noble, 2013.

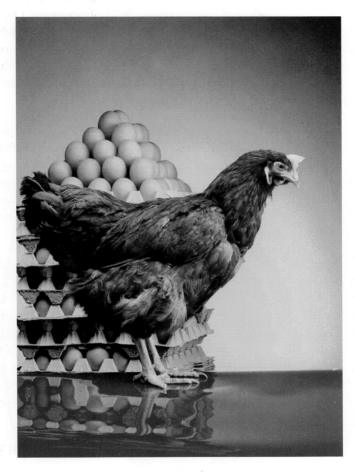

The egg is one of the most versatile ingredients in our diet.

In praise of the egg

O! Eggy Egg my Valentine,

Exquisite shape and tastes divine,

To please my ego - do be mine,

And say that YOU will with me dine.

Ray Noble, 1959

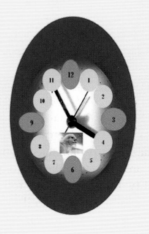

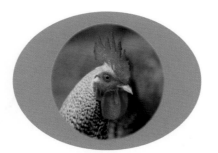

INTRODUCTION

A good beginning makes a good ending

Some 1600 years ago the Greek philosopher Hippocrates stated "Let the food be your medicine and the medicine be your food". In modern terms this can be translated more simply as "You are what you eat". The statement, although not strictly true, still has substantial validity. It is now well recognised that "what we are" is determined by input from a whole range of features that make up our lifestyle and over which we, as individuals, are capable of optional control to a larger or lesser extent. Obvious features include diet, stress, smoking, exercise, medical intervention - to name but a few.

However, diet remains a pivotal determinant and the kitchen can rightly be said to be its control centre. In present day nutrition, the dramatic expansion of food products, both good and bad, their ease of availability, the persuasive nature of marketing and appealing taste are all major players to be considered. Each bears a responsibility for the now all too obvious collective consequences that have led to the well voiced decline in our health and well being. Governmental and professional concerns aimed to turn this tide of self neglect have been, and generally continue to be met by a "canute like" response from a society seemingly hell bent on some sort of self destruction.

Golden Egg

In ancient times we have been told
A goose did lay an egg of gold,
She did produce one every day,
So regular this goose did lay.
But her stupid foolish master
Wanted her to lay them faster,
And he at last the goose did kill,
Gold grist no more came to his mill.
But a strange tale we now unfold,
In California's mines of gold,
There they keep both hens and chickens,
'Mong the gravel scratching pickings.
But hens do find the golden shiner,
Is too heavy for their dinner,
For it they cannot well digest,
As it lies solid in their breast.
Then they are slain and you behold
In their craw the shining gold,
Made up of particles so fine,
The purest gold in all the mine.
Then how happy is the miner,
When he has sweet fowl for dinner,
And he doth find within its craw,
A little golden bonanza.
And in Ontario the hen
Is worthy of the poet's pen,
For she doth well deserve the praise
Bestowed on her for her fine lays.

James McIntyre

It has to be admitted that the situation is not aided by the mixed messages that dominate much of the nutritional information available. Truthful or otherwise, misleading or even basically unsound, the available information is relentless. How often has a dietary recommendation been given due prominence only to be countermanded by subsequent new evidence or findings. Invariably, the consumer is exposed to information overload and unable to know what it all means, that is if much of it has any meaning at all. Widespread confusion is therefore understandable.

Nutritional science is far from simple. It consists of a substantial and complex combination of organic and inorganic dietary groupings. This is made even more complicated by the spread within these groupings of an extensive number of essential nutrients - that is components that the human body is unable to synthesise and so must be included in the diet. Announcements of further discoveries to the already massive list of dietary components seen as having positive inputs to our health and welfare now seem a daily occurrence. Taken in excess, all nutritional components and products of proven benefit can, under certain conditions, also become less than beneficial. Interactions between food components can be negative as well as positive. Taking all this into consideration, it becomes clear that no dietary recommendation can be written in stone. The extent of nutritional data and its interpretation by the public can, in all truth, be said to have reached the point of serious confusion.

A minimum approach being suggested for healthy eating is to abide by three simple principles:

•   variety - a balanced choice from a diverse and well proven list of food components.

Eggs

Eggs! Eggs!
Who lays eggs?
Hens lay eggs.
That I knew!
Only hens?
All birds do!
Only birds?
Not true!
Fish lay eggs
And quite a few!
Birds and fish
And insects, too!
And reptiles and
Amphibians do!
Who's in an egg?
Someone new!
Time to hatch!
Open, you
Eggs! Eggs! Eggs!

Meish Goldish

- moderation - always bear in mind that excessive amounts of any dietary component may be detrimental under certain circumstances and there is a need to maintain a balance between caloric intake and energy expenditure.

- physical activity - regular activity, according to age, is essential for all of us, not only in terms of maintaining an appropriate weight but also for its beneficial effects on metabolic and physiological functions.

In terms of a well tried and established food component, the avian egg has for a long time been passively accepted as possessing an impeccable pedigree, based as it is on a centuries-long nutritional experience. In most instances, justifiable nutritional evidence for this acceptance was sparse to say the least. However, from the beginning of the 20th century, the increasing abilities of scientific analysis enabled the unravelling of nutritional features of the egg at an ever increasing rate. By the 1920's and 30's the egg could be announced as a protective food with positive inputs to health and well being. This reputation was held until well into the 1980's. At this point, public nutritional faith in the egg became increasingly undermined arising from its potential implications in major welfare issues, not least those of coronary and circulatory disorders.

There is now a considerable accumulation of data on the chemical components of the egg and their significant potential in terms of modern nutritional requirements. However, this has been, and still remains, largely within the sphere of the researcher and academic with little such data making it into the public domain. The general public is therefore left to largely rely on generalisations and misinterpretations to assess the worth of the egg as part of their diet. The following is hopefully an appropriate, if belated, effort to reverse this shortcoming.

Q & A

Q.How should eggs be stored?
A. Eggs should be stored in their carton on a shelf in the main body of the refrigerator. Keeping them in the egg compartment on the door will not provide a consistent and cool enough temperature.

Q. How can you tell if an egg is fresh?
A. There is a Best Before date stamped on the end of each carton which indicates freshness. As long as the eggs have been kept refrigerated, this date will reflect approximately how long the eggs will maintain their Grade A freshness and quality. A fresh egg, in its shell, will sink in water while an old egg will float.

It is in no way an attempt to persuade opinion one way or the other with regard to the egg's merit or otherwise in present day health issues. It is an attempt merely to give facts and figures on the range of components that exist within the egg and which can be deemed as nutritionally beneficial. At the very least it is hoped that some degree of interest and understanding will be gleaned about the nutritional diversity of the egg and whether a renewal of nutritional faith is justified or not.

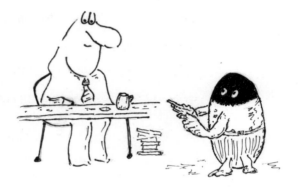

It's very hard to say "NO" to an egg

Did you know that?

❖ Although nearly all animals produce eggs, only some (oviparous) lay them outside their bodies.

❖ There is archaeological evidence dating egg consumption as far back as the Neolithic age.

❖ It was in 1871 that the prototype of the present-day egg carrier was designed.

❖ Before 1871 eggs were stored and carried in baskets lined with hay.

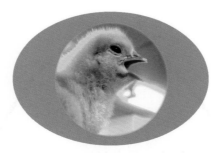

A REPUTATION IN DISPUTE

Health is better than wealth

Human interest in the avian egg is substantial and can be traced back many centuries. The derivation of the word "egg" can also be traced back a long way, coming to prominence in a unique old English form but then overtaken in the 16th. century with the adoption of the word egg from the Nordic language.

Interest in the egg encompasses a range of areas at both amateur and academic levels, for example - art, archaeology, religious and social symbolism, science, natural history, ornithology and nutrition. Such has been the importance of the avian egg to the various facets of our lives that it has given rise to widespread inclusion into everyday conversation. e.g. "a good/bad egg" (somebody of worth/worthless), "all eggs in one basket" (reducing choice), "cannot teach your grandmother to suck eggs" (unacceptable advice), "do not count your chicks before they hatch" (do not anticipate), "addled" (stupid), "over-egged" (to exaggerate), "an egg head" (somebody of intelligence), "walking on eggs" (taking a risk), "cracked" (strange), "egg on your face" (to be embarrassed), - to name but a few!

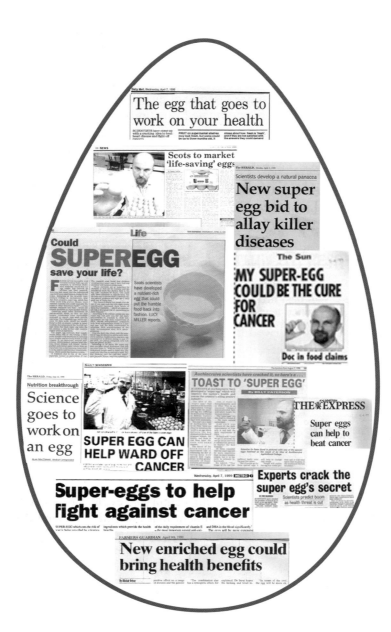

The scientific study of the avian egg was initially confined to egg collection and classification. However, the advance of scientific curiosity and research techniques from the nineteenth century onward has seen the egg, and its contents, come under intense scrutiny and the realisation of its wide range of chemical components and their interrelated functions. The accumulated knowledge to date not only embraces fundamental aspects of the biochemistry and physiology of the avian, and its reproductive processes, but has been exploited to fulfil a host of important roles in various sectors of our lives. Major amongst these has been the role of the egg in our diet.

Almost since the beginning of time, the avian egg has featured as a major, well-tested and trusted component of the human diet. Centuries of consumption of eggs from various species - but nowadays almost wholly confined to the domesticated chicken - have fully validated its range of physical and nutritional merits as prime dietary components and facilitators to our health and well being. Increasing abundance of avian egg supply to succeeding generations has resulted in the diet acceptance of the egg almost without question. No further comment on the egg's dietary worth other than "it is good for us" has ever been necessary. An academic devotee of the egg at the end of the 19th. century went so far as to say that "I think that if required on pain of death to name instantly the most perfect thing in the Universe, I should risk my fate on the bird's egg".

Within the latter part of the 20th. century an event was to occur within our nutritional environment that radically changed the established cosy egg/human dietary relationship - initially for the short term but possibly for the foreseeable future. The event was the sudden recognition that matters health-wise were far from good within the population and getting worse.

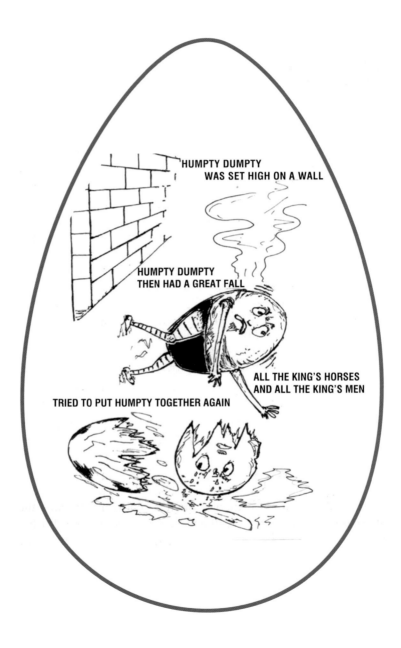

An increasing awareness of an impending pandemic of obesity, accompanied by a selection of directly associated major health problems, was being realised within the public at large and at an increasingly alarming rate. The response from all nutritional sectors was an unleashing of unprecedented actions to unearth and nail the major dietary culprits that could be held responsible for the demise of our health and well being. No component of our diet, from the largest to the smallest, escaped the inquisition. For the guilty parties, verbal and practical retribution was summarily applied. In the case of the egg, its past reputation went for nought and no aspect of its composition was spared from investigation. Matters were found wanting. Adulation to criticism was rapid as evidenced by the removal of eggs from the best market placements to less conspicuous and remoter parts - their place being rapidly filled by glitzy celebs, ready and only too eager to persuade the consumer of the birth of a new and better nutritional dawn. Most significant were recommendations urging restraint in our consumption of eggs as a mainstream component of our daily diet.

The historical establishment of the egg as an unblemished and important part of our diet was largely achieved in the virtual absence of any worthwhile knowledge upon which to make an objective assessment. Under such a scenario, opinion is at the mercy of information from any source and of varied veracity. In the case of the egg, it is now no longer sufficient for its defence to merely rely upon an unquantifiable "goodness" factor. It is time for the egg to make its own case, based on the substantiated nutritional data now available. Such a platform provides the alternative of either an overall acceptance once more or further fuel for detractors to work upon. Inaction at this point in time should certainly not remain an option for those that have the egg's best future at heart.

Egg-related traditions

In Mergentheim, Germany, if someone falls gravely ill, that person ties a white thread around an egg and places it into a fire. If the shell turns black in the flame, death is not far off !!

In Morocco, a woman who has a very young son and is preparing to give birth again keeps an egg close to her during labor. After the birth, the egg is given to the newborn's brother to ensure that the siblings will like each other. But if the egg should happen to be eaten by someone other than the baby's brother, the baby will grow up to hate the mother.

All across Europe, eggs are used to tell fortunes. The most popular method is to carefully pierce the shell and catch drops of the egg white in a glass of water. The shapes that form in the water are examined and interpreted by an unmarried woman who is looking for clues to her future husband's profession. A ship means marriage to a sailor, a shoe means she'll wed a cobbler, and so on.

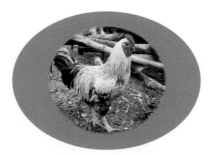

EGG PRODUCING SYSTEMS

You don't have to kill the chicken to get eggs

Eggs are produced via three main types of production systems - cage, barn and free range.

The cage system

These large laying facilities provide hens with an environment of optimal temperature, humidity, feed, water, laying space and security. Even though this housing method may seem to limit the hen's freedom, it is specifically designed to cover all aspects of welfare for the hens in combination with efficiency of production. Indeed, the modern battery cage is designed to satisfy all aspects of the bird's health and well-being. Food is supplied in troughs fitted to the cage fronts and water is supplied automatically. The units have inbuilt climate control to maintain optimal temperature, humidity and ventilation. Computer controlled lighting ensures an optimal day length and light intensity at all times. The cages have sloping mesh floors so that the eggs roll forward out of reach of the birds. In many cases the eggs are collected and packed automatically. Droppings pass through the mesh floors onto boards or moving belts, thereby ensuring that the eggs are clean.

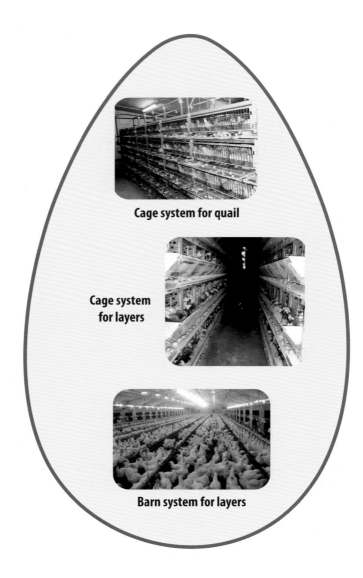

Cage system for quail

Cage system
for layers

Barn system for layers

The cage system is by far the most common method of commercial egg production worldwide. In 2010 the system accounted for around fifty per cent of all eggs produced in the UK.

The barn system

In the barn system the aim is for the hens to have significant freedom of movement. Perches are installed and litter accounts for at least one third of the floor surface thus satisfying requirements for scratching and dust bathing. Linear feeders provide ample space for feeding and there is more than adequate access to drinking facilities. Lighting is again programme controlled to ensure the provision of an optimal day length at all times. At the end of the laying period, the house is completely cleaned and disinfected. Around five per cent of all eggs sold in the UK in 2010 were produced in the barn system of housing.

Free range and organic systems

For eggs to be termed "free range" hens must have continuous daytime access to runs which are mainly covered with vegetation. Housing conditions for the hens must comply with enforceable regulations. The hens have access to nest boxes and perches. Litter should account for at least one third of the accessible ground surface. Although the hens have access to the outside, there are no regulations covering how long they need to be outside, the actual area of the outside or any standards that specifically qualify the use of the term "free range".

The definition of the term organic is wholly dependent on the agency that has defined it and therefore varies from place to place. Organic eggs are produced by hens that receive feed stuffs that have been grown in the complete absence of most conventional pesticides, fungicides, herbicides and commercial fertilisers.

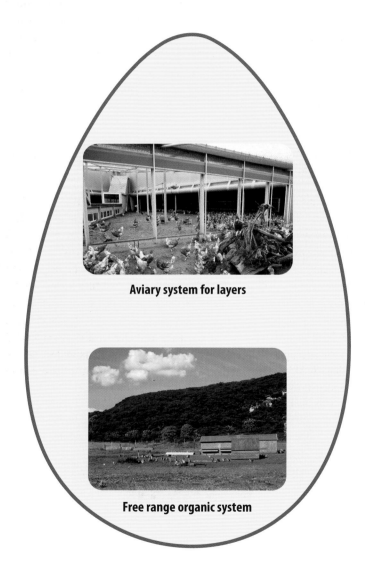

Aviary system for layers

Free range organic system

Organic standards prohibit the use of antibiotics. Although it is not routine practice, the use of antibiotics is allowed under circumstances where there is an absolute necessity for their use to treat sickness. In all conventional systems of egg production, strict controls are in place to ensure the absence of any antibiotic and drug residues in eggs where, for specific reasons, drugs have been supplied in the feed or water. The organic system of egg production should in theory provide no increased risk in terms of consumer safety.

Free range and organic systems accounted for some forty five per cent of all eggs produced in the UK in 2010.

Introduction of the European Union Council Directive (1999/74/EC) effectively banned conventional battery cages in the EU from January 2012. This has led to the development of several alternative non-cage or modified housing systems, such as aviaries and cages that include perches and areas that can provide facilities for foraging, dust bathing and nesting. The move to such systems has aroused considerable doubts from many respected quarters as to any improved outcomes with respect to the health and welfare of the hen and the quality/nutritional safety of the egg. Indeed, there is no general consensus for the superiority of any one housing system over any other regarding food safety and egg quality.

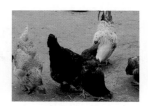

**Table 1. Egg production in EU,
% of total production**

Country	Egg producing system				
	Cage	Barn system	Free-range	Organic	Alternative systems in total
EU-15*, 1996	92	4	4	0	8
EU-15*, 2000	89	5	6	0	11
EU-25*, 2007	75	14	9	2	25
France**	80	3	13	4	20
Spain**	96	2	2	-	4
Germany**	63	22	10	5	37
Netherlands**	46	40	12	2	54
Italy**	79	18	1	2	21
UK**	59	5	35	1	41

*/- number of countries in the EU at that year
**/- data for 2007

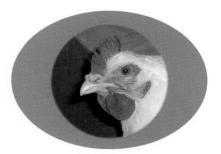

WORLDWIDE EGG PRODUCTION AND CONSUMPTION

Better an egg today than a hen tomorrow

In spite of the doubts being aired in western societies on the health aspects of egg consumption, over the last decade the world's egg production has increased substantially. For example, world production in 2000 was 51.2 million tonnes of eggs, and increased to 59.0; 63.5 and 65.0 million tonnes in 2007, 2010 and 2011 respectively.

Throughout, Asia has accounted for the largest proportion of world production (38.2 million tonnes), with China alone being by far the largest contributor both in Asian and world terms (24.1 million tonnes). Production in North America and Europe, although substantial in population terms, falls far behind that of the Far East. Levels in North and South Americas together is around 13.2 million tonnes and Europe 10.6 million tonnes. By comparison UK production is only some 658 thousand tonnes.

Egg consumption per person ranges widely between countries.

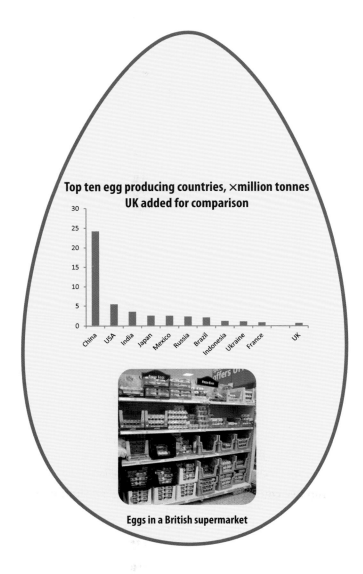

Top ten egg producing countries, ×million tonnes
UK added for comparison

Eggs in a British supermarket

The people of Japan are by far the largest consumers, winning comfortably with an annual consumption of three hundred and forty five eggs per person, or about one per day. India on the other hand comes in at only forty eight eggs per person per year, that is less than one egg per week - clearly a dietary treat to be looked forward to! It is interesting to note that egg consumption in Paraguay increased significantly for the last few years and now it is similar to that in Japan.

The United Kingdom, with an annual consumption of one hundred and eighty three eggs per person is obviously going for the safe option. Whereas in most instances total egg consumption includes a significant proportion of egg products, this is surprisingly far from the case in Mexico.

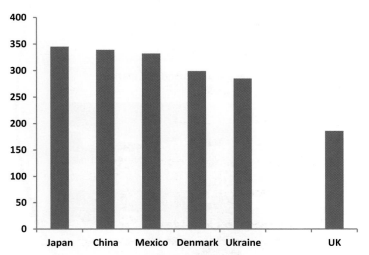

Top five countries with the highest egg consumption, eggs/person/year
*UK added for a comparison

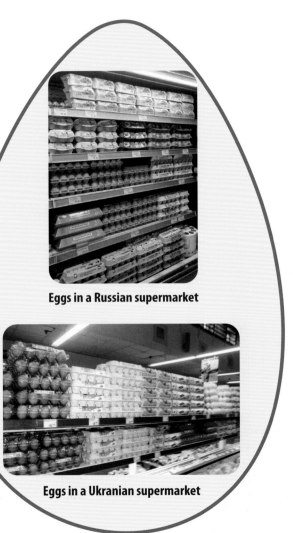

Eggs in a Russian supermarket

Eggs in a Ukranian supermarket

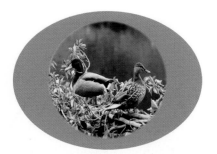

EGG FORMATION

A good beginning makes a good ending

In any discussion of the dietary value of the egg, there is a need to be aware of its reason for existence and general mode of formation. When buying eggs, it is all too easy to forget its primary function, namely to serve as a very successful means of reproduction for the avian. Amongst the most important requirements to achieve this is the nutritional make up of the egg. For this, the developing chick embryo and the emergent chick are extremely well served by the quality and quantity of the nutrients provided. That the egg's nutritional pedigree may not be entirely to human requirements has come as quite a surprise. However, in our contemporary world of the "nutritional microscope", it would be a miracle if no dietary inadequacy or shortcoming was to be found within the egg's nutritional pedigree.

The formation of the egg from its germinal origin to final emergence of an all embracing and sealed nutritional package is a tortuous and fascinating story. The elements of this package, both structural and dietary, are the result of processes of great precision and organisation. In its most simple terms, the egg can be seen as being comprised of three major parts, the yolk, albumen and shell. In quantitative terms, this involves

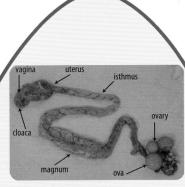

Reproductive organs of the hen

Table 2. Functions of various sections of the hen's oviduct

Section of oviduct	Time egg spends in the section	Functions of section of oviduct
Funnel (infundibulum)	30 min	Receives egg yolk from ovary
Magnum	3 hours	Albumin (white) is secreted and layered around the yolk
Isthmus	1 hour	Inner and outer shell membranes added
Shell gland (uterus)	21 hour	Water is added to swell the albumen - shell calcification and formation of pigmented cuticle
Vagina/cloaca	< 10 min	The egg passes through this section without modification

the transport of substantial quantities of materials across specifically designed membranes at very precise times. In addition to the transport of substantial amounts of materials, their design and synthesis have to be intimately compatible with the requirements for the survival and development of both the embryo and emergent chick.

The starting point of egg formation is a single large ovary which, at sexual maturity, carries thousands of ova (potential yolks) at different stages of development, but each in turn having a potential to initiate the formation of an egg. In spite of the intense rate of egg laying demanded of the modern hen, the total number of eggs produced during a laying lifetime falls far short of ova available. The shedding of a single ovum into a long convoluted tube called the oviduct sees the initiation of egg formation. A combination of continuous rhythmic and fluidic contractions of the oviduct wall propel the ovum/yolk forward. During this, the ovum/yolk is exposed in an orderly manner to a range of well regulated sequential secretions ultimately bound together in a unique structural format to satisfy all the future *in situ* demands of the developing embryo and early chick growth.

The schedule of events from initial ovum engulfment to final egg expulsion takes some twenty four hours. Deposition of the albumen (white) takes place over the first three hour period of the yolk's passage through the oviduct whilst the formation and deposition of the shell takes up almost all the remainder of the egg's passage. With the primary purpose of promoting stability, metabolism and protection of the egg, an extensive range of membranes and structures are incorporated at appropriate times during the twenty four hours of passage. The final act of egg formation before expulsion involves further protection and cosmetic attention through the application of a transparent cuticle and polish to the shell surface.

Did you know that?

❖ The predecessor of the modern chicken, the jungle fowl, had been domesticated in India by 3,200 BC.

❖ The second voyage of Columbus is said to be responsible for the introduction of the domesticated chicken into America.

❖ Egg shells have been used to produce a synthetic ivory for making piano keys. These keys are capable of absorbing oils and moisture which means that the keys are not slippery to the touch.

❖ The duck egg is not suitable for making meringues and soufflés. It lacks the high quality protein present in the chicken's egg and therefore the ability to produce a high quality foam.

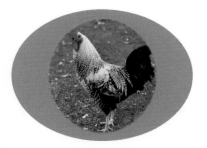

THE LAYING HEN IS AN EGG
PRODUCING FACTORY

All things are easy, that are done willingly

In order to satisfy our demand for eggs, the hen of modern times can be seen as an extreme example of biological exploitation. The demands are not confined purely to a very large and consistent egg output but also include a range of features of a more cosmetic nature appropriate to present day market requirements. Such demands have been secured through extensive physiological manipulation of the entire natural laying process to the extent that there remains little resemblance to that found in the hen's wild counterparts.

The process of egg production in the modern hen is basically as follows. As per normal, the point of ovum shedding to egg laying takes in the region of twenty five hours. Ovulation and the integrated process of egg formation is then induced to start again within about one and a half hours of the previous egg being laid. Eggs will continue to be laid on a twenty four hour basis over a period of some 6-7 days. After a day's rest, ovum release and egg laying starts again. A continuum of this egg laying cycle is then maintained for a period of many months, thereby achieving a total egg output in the region of more than 300 eggs per hen per year.

Did you know that?

❖ Although in nature it is the general rule that the task of incubating the eggs is a shared experience between the male and female, there are some notable exceptions.

❖ After laying her eggs the female emu leaves matters entirely to the male who takes full responsibility for the whole incubation period of some eight weeks, followed by care of the chicks for the whole of the following eighteen months of their life.

❖ In the Emperor penguin the single egg laid by the female is rapidly transferred into the sole care of the male for the full two month period of incubation. The female meanwhile spends her time at sea feeding whilst the male has to exist off reserves of his body fat resulting in the loss of up to forty five percent of his bodyweight.

If commercial requirements allowed, the hen could, after a short break, start the whole cycle again, albeit at a somewhat reduced intensity. Sustaining such an intense egg output, all of an acceptable nutritional quality, clearly imposes a considerable strain on the hen's metabolism and ability to mobilise the required levels of nutrients from its body stores. In the case of the shell, it has been estimated that, over a single laying cycle, the hen achieves an extremely high turnover rate of calcium.

Without doubt intensive breeding has played a major role in developing the hen's ability to conform to modern commercial requirements. In the absence of very strict feeding regimes and environmental controls, this unique egg laying "factory" would clearly be completely unsustainable. The hormonal stimulation of ova release in the hen is controlled naturally by changing light patterns and to achieve egg output and quality, this feature is maximally exploited through the continuous imposition of dark/light sequencing patterns. Extreme attention is paid to all quantitative and qualitative aspects of the diet. Environmentally controlled housing to ensure the hen's well being and comfort completes the hen's pattern of existence.

Having satisfied all the required features for output, the egg must also pass a whole series of physical parameters seen as essential for market acceptance. In the main these embrace aspects of little relevance to nutritional quality and more to satisfy a modern marketing obsession for a cosmetic appeal. Thus, for example, fresh eggs must be free from extraneous odour, of highly uniform shape and size, the shell to be of an unblemished uniform colour, good texture, sound, unstained and with an undamaged polished cuticle, the albumen must be translucent, limpid and of a gelatinous consistency and the yolk must be free from blemish, translucent, centrally

Did you know that?

❖ Initially the hen has two functional ovaries but the right one rapidly regresses leaving egg production solely reliant upon the left ovary.

❖ Removal of a functional left ovary results in the right ovary developing into a testis (male gonad). This sex reversed bird can produce spermatozoa.

❖ Most birds lay eggs of a similar shape to that of the hen. Long pointed eggs are a feature of sea birds which nest on cliff ledges. If knocked out of the nest they will roll in a circle affording some protection against falling off.

❖ Pointed eggs are also laid by birds that lay large numbers as they take up less space in the nest and can be covered more easily by the sitting partner.

placed and not moving away from the centre of the egg during rotation. Bearing in mind that it is the nutritional content and quality for which the egg is being sold, then it might seriously be suggested that purchase would be little harmed by less attention to several of such parameters.

However, appearance and presentation are matters of dominating importance in the present day market and are being used increasingly as a persuasive, if sometimes illogical, means for influencing customer preference. In this respect the egg has been very much a victim of consumer preferences. In spite of the best nutritional efforts by the hen to provide on our behalf a good product, in the contemporary food market reliance on nutritional benefits alone is no longer an option.

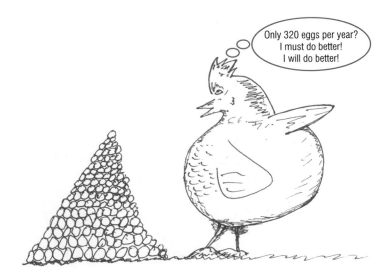

Did you know that?

❖ Alligators, crocodiles, snakes, lizards and a range of other reptiles indulge in what is known as temperature dependant reproduction. This means that the sex of the hatchling is determined by the incubation temperature or any temperature changes experienced during incubation.

❖ For the alligator and crocodile, increasing the temperature of incubation increases the proportion of male offspring up to 100% of the hatch.

❖ Reducing incubation temperature increases the proportion of females up to 100%. For alligators and crocodiles this is the sole determinant of the hatchling's sex.

❖ Lizards, snakes etc. have a choice of either temperature dependant sex or, as for the human and the vast majority of animals, chromosomal sex.

❖ The avian may have access to temperature sex determination.

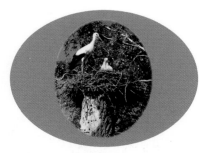

EGG STRUCTURE

".............an architectural marvel"

The internal elements of the egg are organised and arranged in an interdependent order specifically designed to satisfy its biological function of embryo development. The nutrients are enclosed within a well structured and fortified coat – the shell – whose protective function to the contents is supplemented by the elasticity of the albumen. In gross terms the egg can be considered to be divided between three major components, some sixty per cent albumen, thirty per cent yolk and around ten per cent shell. Although under natural conditions these proportions may vary significantly, this is much less likely under highly controlled modern intensive production systems.

The almost spherical yellow/orange yolk is enclosed within an elastic membrane and is centrally suspended by two bands of protein (chalazae) attached to the pointed and blunt ends of the shell. Appearances are deceptive. The yolk is not homogeneous. It is composed of a series of alternating narrower white and much broader yellow layers. The white layers account for only around two per cent of total yolk material and display a high water content compared to the fat (lipid) rich and highly pigmented yellow layers. Yolk

Did you know that?

❖ The egg provides essential ingredients for a wide range of products (cheese making, vaccines, throat lozenges, eye drops, lens decontaminates, shampoos, skin treatments, soaps, to name but a few).

❖ Eggs are processed into many refrigerated formats (liquid, frozen pulp, dried whole egg, yolk or white).

❖ Speciality egg products include whole egg hard-boiled, peeled, chopped, frozen, fried and poached, scrambled and omelette mix and ready whites.

❖ The physical properties of the egg (foaming, coagulation, emulsification, homogenisation) are essential to cooking.

colour is open to significant variation, from a pale yellow to a dark orange. Yolk colour is of major importance to the consumer, largely for subjective cosmetic reasons as opposed to any obvious inherent nutritional value. As the colour is extremely sensitive to plant pigments (carotenoids) within the diet and to satisfy differing consumer demands, much attention is paid to its natural and/or artificial presence in feeding programmes. Enclosing the yolk is a thin pliable envelope known as the yolk vitelline membrane.

Surrounding the yolk is the translucent fluid known as the albumen but which, based on its change following coagulation, is commonly referred to as the "white". The albumen accounts for some sixty per cent of total egg weight. As in the case of the yolk, the albumen is also distinctively layered. In contrast to the yolk, the relative proportions of the three component layers may vary significantly but in general equate to some seventeen, fifty eight and twenty three per cent respectively for the inner, middle and outer layers. By attachment of the albumen to sections of the shell, it is able to act as a protective sac that cushions the yolk from physical damage. Two membranes exist between the albumen and the shell, one surrounding the albumen and the other firmly attached and fully covering the inner surface wall of the shell. At the blunt end of the egg there is an air space (air cell).

Finally there is the shell itself, composed almost wholly of calcium carbonate, permeated by a myriad of pores and clothed by a very thin transparent protein coating, the cuticle. Although the major property of the shell is commonly seen as its rigidity and therefore solely for the cohesion and protection of the egg, its structure plays a significant role in maintaining egg quality by preventing microbial entry and the control of moisture loss. A feature of the cuticle is its inherent pigmentation which in commercial terms is a very

Did you know that?

❖ A kiwi's egg can account for about 20 per cent of the parent's body weight just before laying. This is the largest egg-to-body weight ratio of any bird.

❖ Eggs of the Royal Albatross take 79 days to hatch. It is the longest incubation period for an egg.

❖ All birds are divided into two major groups, Precocial and Altricial birds:

1. Precocial birds: down-covered chicks, such as domestic chickens, turkeys, geese, ducks and gulls, hatch ready to move around, eat on their own and leave the nest if necessary.

2. Altricial birds such as owls, woodpeckers, and most songbirds, are hatched naked, blind, and helpless. They need lots of care from parents to survive.

important function. In the UK the aesthetic appeal of brown eggs is dominant and is of massive market significance. Not so in the rest of Europe or America where white is preferred. As in the case of the yolk, shell colour is of aesthetic appeal only with no meaningful reference to the egg's nutritional worth.

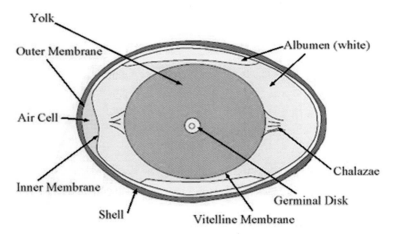

Structure of the egg

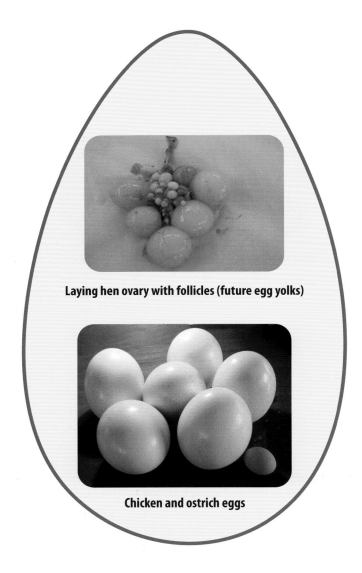

Laying hen ovary with follicles (future egg yolks)

Chicken and ostrich eggs

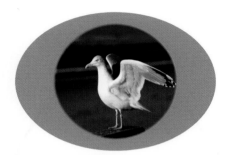

GENERAL NUTRITIVE VALUE OF THE EGG

"...the egg is an Aladdin's Cave of nutrients"

In common with all animal tissues, the contents of the egg consists predominantly of water. Present as solids are fats (lipids to give them their scientific title), proteins, carbohydrates, minerals and vitamins. Lipids and proteins predominate. In both absolute and proportional terms all the components are open to manipulation, mainly through the diet but to some extent through genetic and environmental influences.

Whereas the protein is evenly distributed between both the albumen and the yolk, lipids are almost wholly confined to the yolk. Minerals and vitamins are also distributed throughout both the albumen and yolk. In the case of the minerals, distribution is largely determined by their functional association with organic compounds, leaving only a small proportion in free inorganic form. Although of no direct nutritional value, the egg's high water content is of a significant indirect importance through its role in preserving the chemical integrity of the solubilized nutrients. Its role in temperature control protects the proteins from irreversible denaturation whilst, by ensuring contact

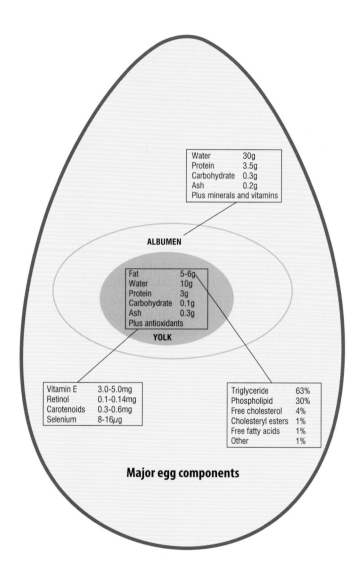

Water	30g
Protein	3.5g
Carbohydrate	0.3g
Ash	0.2g
Plus minerals and vitamins	

ALBUMEN

Fat	5-6g
Water	10g
Protein	3g
Carbohydrate	0.1g
Ash	0.3g
Plus antioxidants	

YOLK

Vitamin E	3.0-5.0mg
Retinol	0.1-0.14mg
Carotenoids	0.3-0.6mg
Selenium	8-16μg

Triglyceride	63%
Phospholipid	30%
Free cholesterol	4%
Cholesteryl esters	1%
Free fatty acids	1%
Other	1%

Major egg components

between the dissolved components, destructive interacting reactions are largely avoided or reduced.

The egg's nutritional components are far from simple in their chemistry, a feature that is made very much more complicated by intricate interlocking associations between individual components and chemical groupings. There is, therefore, no simple or elementary description that can be applied to the composition of the egg. It is this that has provided the egg's major fascination and challenge over the centuries.

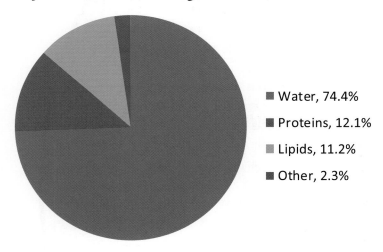

■ Water, 74.4%

■ Proteins, 12.1%

■ Lipids, 11.2%

■ Other, 2.3%

Basic egg composition

Q & A

Q. How often does a hen lay an egg?
A. The entire time from ovulation to laying is about 25 hours. After about 30 minutes the process starts again.

Q. What is the source of yolk colour?
A. Yolk colour in eggs is directly linked to the diet of the hens and determined by natural pigments known as carotenoids. Main sources of the carotenoids are maize and green vegetation.

Q. Why is the egg white sometimes cloudy?
A. Cloudiness of raw white is due to the natural presence of carbon dioxide which has not had time to escape through the shell and is an indication of a very fresh egg. As an egg ages, the carbon dioxide escapes via the shell and the egg white becomes more transparent.

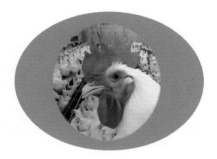

PROTEINS

The way to a man's heart is through his stomach

Proteins are a major basic building block of the human body, accounting for some sixteen per cent of total body weight. As well as being the major components of important organs and tissues, proteins play an essential role in determining the structure and intimate functioning of all cells, for example through their presence in enzymes, hormones and neurotransmitters. In more general terms, they are key elements for protection against bacterial and viral invasion, nutrient absorption and transport and overall body development. In fact there is virtually no part of bodily function and well being that does not have a heavy reliance on, or input from, proteins.

Although our bodies are good at recycling proteins, there is little capacity for their storage. Thus the absence or severe reduction of dietary protein intake sees a rapid breakdown of muscle tissue. It is therefore essential to health and well-being to maintain an adequate dietary protein supply, an ability to break it down into smaller components and, following intestinal absorption, resynthesis of proteins required to sustain our bodily structures.

Did you know that?

❖ The egg has a long and distinguished association with painting as an essential ingredient to the fast-drying medium known as tempera.

❖ Its use in the art world goes back to ancient Greek and Roman times and in the early Renaissance period of the 15th. century it was the most popular form of painting throughout Europe.

❖ It was used by virtually every famous painter of the time, Duccio, Giotto, Fra Angelico, Ghirlandaio, Mamtegna, and Botticelli.

❖ Late renaissance artists such as Michelangelo and Leonardo da Vinci were well versed in its use. In 1901 The Society of Tempera Painters was founded in London for the revival of tempera use.

The amount of protein required to be consumed as part of a nutritionally adequate diet is dependent on a range of features, major amongst them being age, body mass and activity level. It is generally accepted that for the average healthy person weighing around 60 - 80 kg, daily protein intake should be of the order of 48 - 64 grams. For active groups such as athletes, the required level needs to be higher to take into account increases in protein breakdown, the need for subsequent body repair and loss of body fluids.

A single 60 gram egg contains some 6 gram of protein distributed between the egg white (3.6 gram) and, not always appreciated, the egg yolk (2.7 gram). Consumption of a single egg thus provides more than ten per cent of the protein requirement of the average adult.

The basic structure of proteins is comprised of smaller units known as amino acids. There are twenty one amino acids which are divisible into two groups, nine essential and twelve non-essential. The essential acids are unable to be synthesised within the body and thus must be wholly present in the diet. Therefore the nutritional value of any protein source is dependent upon the composition and content of the essential amino acids and their availability. In this respect egg protein contains all the essential amino acids in the correct proportions required by the body for optimum growth and maintenance.

Indeed, egg protein outperforms all other proteins from either animal or plant sources and therefore is unrivaled in suiting human dietary requirements. It is also important to underline that egg protein is easily digested and absorbed. It is notable that the quality of egg protein is routinely used as the standard against which the nutritional qualities of all other proteins are measured.

Did you know that?

❖ During the middle ages whole egg and it's ingredients were widely used as an essential ingredient of specific building materials, in particular for water resistance, appearance and adherence/ setting time of the "concrete".

❖ Most notable structures in which the egg and it's components played an important role are the construction of the Moscow Kremlin (built 16th.-17th. centuries) and one of Prague's most impressive sights, the Charles Bridge built between 1347 and 1402, where the master builders mixed egg into the mortar to strengthen bonding.

In terms of the combination of features for ease of digestion, tissue incorporation/repair and unrivaled amino acid quality, egg protein is recognised throughout all major feed and nutritional sectors in the world as the gold standard.

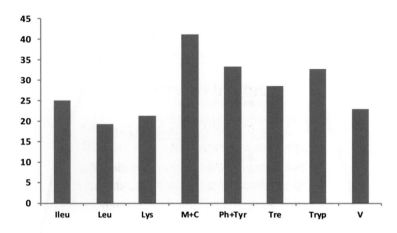

Essential amino acids supplied by a single egg, % of daily requirement

(Ileu = isoleucine; Leu = leucine; Lys = lysine; M+C = methionine + cystine; Ph+Tyr = phenylalanine+tyrosine; Tre = threonine; Tryp = tryptophan; V = valine)

UNDERSTANDING LIPIDS (1)

❖ Extensive permutations and combinations occur between the basic lipid components and can be numbered in the hundreds, all with their own distinctive metabolic and nutritional functions.

❖ This situation is further complicated by protein/lipid complexing that has to occur for the lipid dissolution/solubilisation required for dietary uptake and usage.

❖ Meaningful analytical fractionation of the lipids requires the intervention of highly sophisticated instrumentation.

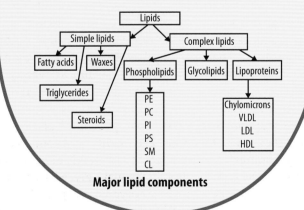

Major lipid components

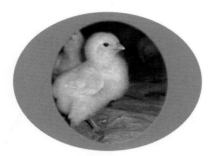

LIPIDS

"...friend or foe?..."

The term lipid is used to cover a wide range of complex substances that are insoluble in water but soluble in organic solvents. Any discussion of fat (lipid) in terms of nutrition and diet is no longer a simple matter. Long gone are the days when to maintain a healthy lifestyle, all that was required was to eat as little fat as possible. Nowadays the terms "good fat" and "bad fat" and their nutritional roles in our health and well being are daily features of heated discussion. However, that some fats are an essential part of our daily diet is now accepted without question. The term lipid embraces a vast range of chemical components, their composition almost wholly able to be described by three common elements - carbon, hydrogen and oxygen - in combinations and permutations which enable them to be segregated into distinctive groupings and families, each with their own functions and bodily distributions. The principle groupings are comprised of fatty acids either alone or chemically linked to an alcohol, in the main glycerol, and which in turn may be combined with other organic compounds to form a host of derived complexes. With the major components being fatty acids, the term lipid may simply be described as "fatty acids and their derivatives".

UNDERSTANDING LIPIDS (2)

❖ Lipids are more commonly referred to as fat, lipid is their scientific term.

❖ They are a major and essential component of our diet and are insoluble in water.

❖ They are almost entirely made up of carbon, hydrogen and oxygen with only a marginal presence of other elements, for example phosphorus. The basic component of all lipids is a group of compounds known as fatty acids.

❖ Their structural characteristic is a backbone of regular carbon/hydrogen units in combinations ranging from two to twenty six units in length. The most abundant dietary fatty acids, and also the most important in terms of the diet, are the fatty acids ranging from 14 to 22 carbon/hydrogen units.

❖ The terminal structure of the fatty acids is such that they are able to link with other chemical entities in such a way that give rise to the major distinctive classes/ groupings that together characterise a lipid.

An essential feature to lipid existence and function in an aqueous environment is solubilisation. This is achieved by lipid interaction with proteins to form complexes known as lipoproteins. As a result of the extensive abilities to combine, permutate and interact, the natural lipid mix encountered within the egg and all animal tissues presents a very intricate picture.

The average sixty gram egg contains approximately six grams of lipid within its yolk. In order to provide this to the egg on a daily basis, both the liver and blood plasma of the hen become engorged with lipid. Three components, triglycerides, phospholipids and cholesterol dominate the lipid composition of the yolk and therefore, in turn, its nutritional quality. For the triglycerides and phospholipids, nutritional quality is determined by the attached fatty acids; cholesterol basically stands alone. Dietary fat intake and its quality has become a major focus of our contemporary lifestyle, in particular with respect to the role of animal derived fats. With its obvious display of a high fat content in a single visually prominent compartment, namely the yolk, the egg has inevitably been drawn into the whole controversy of fat intake and quality.

Evaluation of lipid quality in terms of health and well being primarily involves two major lipid components, the fatty acids and cholesterol. The role of both in the aetiology of cardiovascular disease and other human ailments still remains a highly controversial issue. Based largely upon the visual awareness of the significant lipid presence in the yolk, it has become the general opinion that egg consumption should be treated with great suspicion in terms of a healthy lifestyle.

In other animal products, a significant proportion of the total fat content lies well shielded from view hidden away within

UNDERSTANDING LIPIDS (3)

❖ Fatty acids in free form have a minimal presence in the diet and exist almost entirely bound or linked to other chemical groupings. The resulting formats enable division into distinct classes.

❖ The major of these are:

(i) the triglycerides which have 3 fatty acids attached to the alcohol-glycerol. Far less common are diglycerides (2 fatty acids attached) and monoglycerides (1 fatty acid attached).

(ii) the phosholipids which have 2 fatty acids attached to the glycerol, the third attachment point being taken by phosphoric acid onto which is joined one of a selection of nutritional compounds called bases (e.g. choline, serine, etc.).

(iii) free cholesterol which is also composed of carbon, hydrogen and oxygen but in contrast to the fatty acids, takes the form of a multiple ring structure. Cholesterol can also have a fatty acid attached and it is then referred to as a cholesterol ester.

❖ Within the lipid pool further components may exist e.g. carotenoids, alcohol, pigments, but in gross terms are of minimal importance.

the structural elements of the tissues. In terms of the nutritional quality, that of the egg far outstrips that of almost all other commonly consumed animal fats e.g. bovine products being a worst case example and marine fish an example of faultless quality. With regard to total fat intake, the consumption of a single 60g egg per day would only contribute 4-5 per cent of the total U.K. recommended daily intake. Although basic dietary fat composition remains irrefutable, persuasive arguments in terms of dietary acceptance or rejection abound. In this respect the egg has received more than its fair share of attention.

It was only in the 1960's that the inherent water insolubility of lipids, which had precluded any truly meaningful analytical data to be obtained, was finally overcome by the development of unique instrumentation. By chance, the ensuing rapid evolution in lipid analytical abilities occurred at the same time that concerns for major aspects of our health and well being were being raised.

It is not by accident therefore that lipids became, and still remain, a very significant part of intense and diverse interpretations on the relationship between diet and health. Indeed, such discussion may be considered to have reached the point of an obsession, an obsession which is still largely undermining the desire from responsible quarters for balanced information and interpretation.

UNDERSTANDING LIPIDS (4)

❖ The most important nutritional feature of the fatty acids is their state of "unsaturation". They are divided into saturated and unsaturated forms.

❖ Saturated fatty acids are those where all the carbon/hydrogen units of the chain are complete. Unsaturated fatty acids are those where one or more of the carbon/hydrogen units of the chain are not complete, leaving "gaps" referred analytically as double bonds.

❖ The presence of double bonds confers a highly significant nutritional difference on the fatty acids, those with double bonds (the unsaturates) fulfilling a wide range of essential dietary requirements and therefore of major health benefit whilst those with no double bonds (the saturates) lack any dietary essentiality. Much is made dietarily of this difference, excess intake of the saturates being seen as unfavourable and the intake of the unsaturates, in particular the polyunsaturates, as highly favourable.

❖ Examples of saturates are palmitic and stearic acids and are very common to our diet; examples of polyunsaturates are linoleic and linolenic acids and are mostly confined to specific components of our diet.

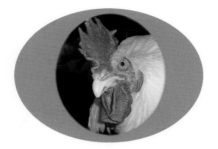

FATTY ACIDS AND CHOLESTEROL

The devil is not so black as he is painted

Fatty acids are the major constituents of lipids within the tissues and fluids of our body. Their essentiality to the structure and function of all tissue and cell functions is well documented. Fatty acids are therefore indispensable to our existence. In terms of health and well being, fatty acids are divisible into three major groups - saturated, monounsaturated and polyunsaturated with the latter further divided into omega-6 and omega-3 components. In simple nutritional terms, the three groups are routinely referred to respectively as bad, neutral and good. This arbitrary delineation of the fatty acids, simple as it may be, is unhelpful.

In spite of the best reasons for introducing such terminology, it is open to extensive misinterpretation. In nutrition, the term "bad fatty acids" is used virtually exclusively in reference to the saturates whose origins in the body arise from both tissue synthesis and dietary supply. However, the saturates do have their own uniquely essential part to play in cell and tissue function. It is only under circumstances of dietary excess that the saturates become unbalanced in their action implicated in adverse physiological effects.

UNDERSTANDING LIPIDS (5)

❖ Linoleic and linolenic acids are the parents for two distinct series of essential acids, respectively known as the omega-6 and omega-3 polyunsaturates

❖ The series are more scientifically referred to as the (n-6) and (n-3) acids

❖ The fatty acid derivatives are achieved by the elongating of the carbon chain by two carbon atoms at a time and the introduction of further double bonds. The prescribed pattern of synthesis is common to both series.

❖ The biological conversion of linoleic and linolenic acids to the members of the series can be described as:

18:2 (n-6)[linoleic acid] → 18:3(n-6) → 20:4(n-6) [arachidonic acid].

18:3(n-3)[linolenic acid] → 20:5(n-3)[eicosapentaenoic acid] → 22:6(n-3) [docosahexaenoic acid]

❖ Abbreviations are also commonly used for each of the major fatty acid components - respectively LA, alpha LNA, AA, EPA and DHA

The term "good" fatty acids is used in reference to the polyunsaturates which uniquely cannot be synthesised by the body and have to be supplied solely by the diet. The term "good" may also be used guardedly in reference to the monounsaturated fatty acids but whose origins, like the saturates, are both by synthesis and the diet.

A simple but far better division of the fatty acids is that used in scientific descriptions, namely essential for the polyunsaturates and non-essential for the remainder. This simple description more adequately embodies both the origins and functional differences between the fatty acids.

With respect to nutrition, non essential fatty acids can be said to be confined to far more basic roles in lipid function and cell structure. In general, the major roles for the non essential fatty acids may be described as facilitators to maintain a lipid presence and cell integrity. By comparison, the polyunsaturates are the activators with involvements in a wide range of highly specific metabolic functions essential to health and well being - for example essential roles in brain function, neurotransmission, immune function, hormone (prostaglandin) synthesis, male reproduction and nutrient metabolism at cellular level.

Fatty acids not only function as individuals within a very extensive and active group of bodily components but also equally through integral associations with other metabolites. Their highly complex roles defy any simple description that is anywhere near capable of differentiation in simple terms of chemistry or function.

The average chicken's egg contains some 5 g of lipid which is almost wholly confined to the yolk. Table 3 shows the lipid

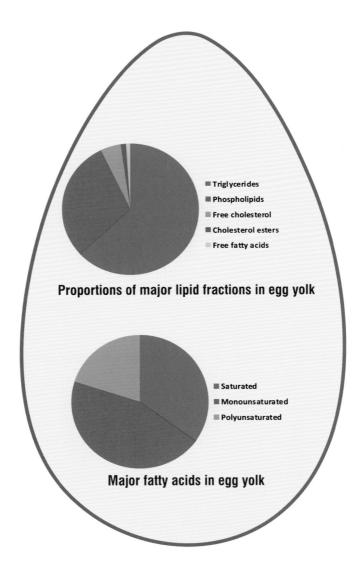

Proportions of major lipid fractions in egg yolk

- Triglycerides
- Phospholipids
- Free cholesterol
- Cholesterol esters
- Free fatty acids

Major fatty acids in egg yolk

- Saturated
- Monounsaturated
- Polyunsaturated

composition of an average egg expressed in terms of the major parameters used in the assessment of lipids for dietary quality. In terms of the proportion of total and individual polyunsaturated fatty acids, those of the yolk compare favourably or even exceed those of a wide range of highly acceptable animal products, including the range of standard margarines in which the total polyunsaturates comprise 20-25 per cent of total fatty acids. Thus in combination with a high level of oleic acid, the yolk is predominately unsaturated.

With a polyunsaturated to saturated fatty acid ratio of 0.6, the yolk clearly exceeds the nutritional target figure for healthy eating. With a total n-6:n-3 polyunsaturated fatty acid ratio of about 8:1, the yolk lipid only just fails to meet the 6:1 ratio suggested as required to take into account the contemporary dietary metabolic imbalance between the two acids. As discussed later, this shortfall in n-3 provision is open to simple remedy.

Over the years, our dietary intake of cholesterol via the egg has been the target for extensive comment, almost all of which has been adverse. The level of cholesterol in the egg has been, and still remains, a major focus of dietary discussion. As the result of a major involvement of cholesterol in the chemistry of cardio-vascular and other circulatory disorders, it has become a feature of opinion to treat all dietary cholesterol sources with great caution.

Although the diet has been seen as the major source of cholesterol, the tissues, in particular the liver, are of equal or of more importance. Levels of cholesterol in the body are regulated by a play off between tissue synthesis and dietary

Table 3. Cholesterol and fatty acid levels in egg lipids, %

Lipids	Value
Cholesterol[1]	4.5
Saturated fatty acids[2]	35
Mono-unsaturated fatty acids[2]	45
Polyunsaturated fatty acids (PUFAs)[2]	
Linoleic	16
Alpha-linolenic	1
C20+C22 PUFAs	3
Total PUFAs	20
Polyunsaturated:saturated fatty acid (P:S) ratio:	
UK dietary recommendation	0.45
Egg	0.59
n6:n3 PUFAs ratio:	
UK dietary recommendation	6
Egg	8

[1] proportion by weight % of total lipid
[2] proportion by weight % of total fatty acids

supply. Thus tissue production of cholesterol increases when dietary sources are reduced and vice versa.

Under normal situations, this mechanism determines the maintenance of a relative steady state for the concentration of cholesterol in the circulation and tissues. Scientific evidence now available opines that for the average healthy individual under normal nutritional circumstances, diet is not the major determinant of blood cholesterol levels and contributor to circulatory problems. At worst, the dietary intake of cholesterol exerts a minimal effect on lasting blood cholesterol levels and is of reduced clinical significance.

However, the finding that the major source of cholesterol within our circulation and tissues arises from bodily synthesis and not through the diet has, to a large extent, failed to allay public and even professional perceptions on the nutritional advocacy of egg consumption and its cholesterol delivery.

In relative terms, the percentage of cholesterol in yolk/ egg lipid is comparable to the lipids of most other animal products. However, in absolute terms the amount of cholesterol supplied by a single egg (about 200-250 mg) has to be considered as high. The feature has been made even worse by the way in which the level of cholesterol has been interpreted, per unit weight of egg or per unit weight of yolk. The fact remains that weight for weight of total lipid there is no difference in the cholesterol level in the whole egg and lipids of other animal products.

Numerous attempts have been made to reduce the level of cholesterol in the egg yolk, ranging from the manipulation of dietary components, genetic selection and through to the administration of drugs. Without doubt, and in spite of all

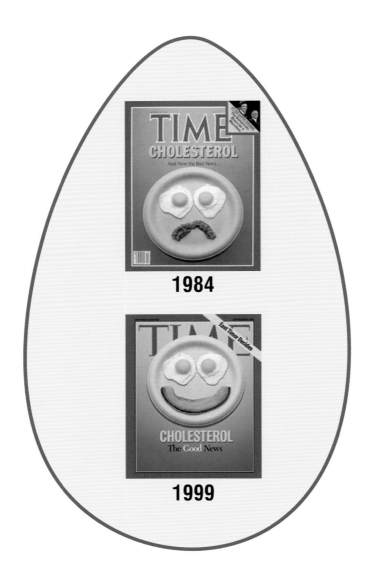

these attempts, egg yolk cholesterol levels have proved to be resistant to any change. Based on in-depth understanding of the processes involved in egg yolk formation, it is now doubtful whether further pursuance of this goal is a worthwhile proposition.

In spite of all the evidence to date, there continue to be claims of success in producing a low cholesterol egg. However, such statements are highly questionable and instill little confidence being based on, for example, the production of eggs with smaller yolk size and the use of analytical techniques that for some reason give answers that are lower than obtained by standard methodologies. Various extractive technologies for the reduction of cholesterol levels in yolk preparations have been devised. However, most of these for one reason or another (for example expense and impracticality) are of little commercial value. Whilst they may reduce the level of cholesterol in the yolk extract, they also remove many other lipid components and therefore limit nutritional benefits.

Taking note of all the evidence, the egg could be considered to present no greater risk to health than many major components of our daily diet. In the light of the data on the relationship between dietary cholesterol intake and bodily synthesis, contemporary concerns on the potential health risks from cholesterol levels in the egg now seem to have gone into reverse. It is therefore joining the all too common feature in recommendations on diet and health that the persuasive "do's" of today become so easily the "don't's" of tomorrow - or vice versa.

In our present health obsessed society, discussion on the role of the egg's cholesterol content has been an over-riding

Bizarre things that people do with eggs

The World Egg Throwing Championship

This took place in Lincolnshire, England in June, 2012. The championship is comprised of five disciplines; Egg Throwing, Egg Static Relay, Egg Target Throwing, Russian Egg Roulette and Egg Trebuchet Challenge.

In accordance with rules, Egg Throwing comprises two-person teams, the winner being the team that can throw and catch an egg over the greatest distance. The team members start off 10 metres apart. After each throw each member moves further apart.

Teams from as far apart as Germany and South Africa had gathered for the event. The Dutch won the distance-throwing event by tossing a raw egg 40m but failed to break their own record of 63.2m.

The sport dates back to 1322 when a newly appointed local Abbot ensured church attendance by providing each peasant with an egg. However, when the local river flooded that year, the monks were forced to hurl the eggs over to the waiting peasants who were unable to attend the service.

feature in decisions on the egg's nutritional role. Present data may not have gone so far as to completely expunge the past but it has been more than sufficient for the egg to now take some comfort. As in all aspects of nutrition, the role of any single component must be kept in balance with all others. This applies as much to cholesterol as to anything else.

Positive references to an essential need for cholesterol rarely features in any dietary discussions. The fact is that cholesterol is a vital, functional part of all cells and tissues where it is integral to a raft of structural and regulatory processes. For instance, the maintenance of cell membrane fluidity, so essential for the passage and excretion and metabolites, brain and nerve function, hormone production, vitamin D synthesis and immune function to name but a few.

Can it now be stated that for the egg and its lipid content the demons, which for so long have haunted acceptance, have been exorcised? If so, can the egg now come out of its semi-exclusion zone and once more take its place as a guilt-free component of our daily diet? Unfortunately the truism of the statement that "the evil that men do lives after them, the good is often interned with their bones" may have resonance with the saga of the egg and its lipid content.

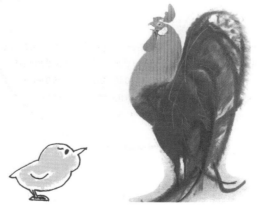

Did you know that?

❖ UK scientists have developed genetically modified chickens capable of laying eggs containing proteins central to manufacture of cancer-fighting drugs.

❖ The breakthrough was announced by the same research centre that created the cloned sheep Dolly. The Roslin Institute, near Edinburgh, claims to have produced five generations of birds that can produce useful levels of life-saving proteins in egg whites.

❖ Some of the birds have been engineered to lay eggs that contain antibodies with potential for treating malignant melanoma, a form of skin cancer.

❖ Other teams produced the human protein interferon and antibodies in eggs to prevent the replication of viruses in cells.

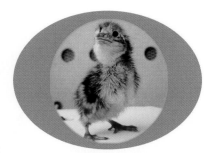

DESIGNER EGGS WITH OMEGA-3 FATTY ACIDS

There is no accounting for taste

Well before the advent of sophisticated technology and the ability to unravel the complexities of lipids and their associated fatty acid components, it became recognised that certain fatty acids played an essential role in the maintenance of our health and well being. It is now fully recognised that omega-6 and omega-3 polyunsaturated fatty acids, which have to be supplied via the diet, are of major importance.

Collectively the list of physiological, structural and metabolic problems arising from their absence or their marginal presence in the diet encompasses an array of roles, from cell and tissue structure and function to essential controls over a wide range of metabolic activities.

Examples of their importance to major tissues are their well proven essentiality for the development and function of the brain, nervous tissues, vision and sperm production. Awareness of the functional importance of the essential fatty acids to our health dates from the 1930's. The ensuing and presently on-going accumulation of data on their involvements in so many

Table 4. Major polyunsaturated fatty acids in egg lipids, %

	Linoleic	Alpha-linolenic	Arachi-donic	Docosa-hexaenoic
Chicken, commercial	15	1	2	1
Chicken, free -range	6	3	2	3
Turkey, commercial	14	1	2	1
Quail, commercial	14	1	1	<1
Duck, commercial	8	<1	10	1
Duck, wild	7	<1	12	4
Pheasant, commercial	16	2	1	1
Pheasant, wild	9	27	1	1
Ostrich, commercial	9	3	<1	<1
Ostrich, wild	9	22	1	<1
Alligator, wild	6	4	4	5

aspects of our metabolism defines their major nutritional importance. Initial attention was focused on those fatty acids of the omega-6 series and therefore products containing enhanced levels of the major omega-6 acid (linoleic acid) became common place and still largely remain so.

The realisation that the fatty acids of the omega-3 series were the equal to, or even more important than, those of the omega-6 series has been slow to come about. Indeed, the very high omega-6/omega-3 ratios present in many of the modified components of our diet is being increasingly recognised as potentially counter-productive in health terms. It is now accepted that to be effective in health terms, a more equal balance between the two groups of omega acids has to be achieved.

The accumulated evidence of a unique essentiality for the omega-3 fatty acids to so many important aspects of our health has appropriately led to a deliberate enhancement within major dietary items. Out of this has arisen the concept of an omega-3 enhanced egg.

The modern hen which is maintained in a stable environment, is of high reproductive capacity and is receiving a sufficiency of a well designed diet, will produce an abundance of eggs of a quite uniform lipid quality. Small differences in both yolk lipid composition and fatty acid quality are observed between strains and breeds and birds of different ages. However, when compared with eggs from wild birds or more naturally maintained hens, there are marked divergences in fatty acid composition, in particular in the range of unsaturated components.

As can be seen from Table 4, eggs from intensive or farmed production systems display high levels of fatty

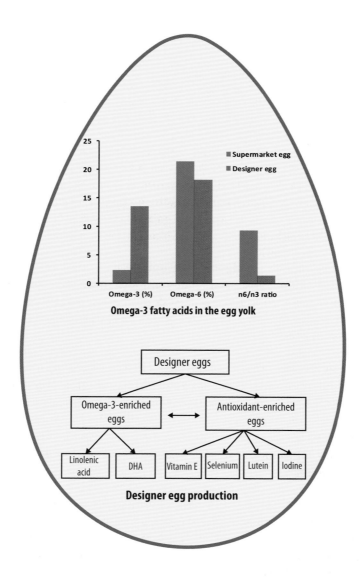

Omega-3 fatty acids in the egg yolk

Designer egg production

acids belonging to the n-6 series, in particular linoleic acid, and contrast sharply with eggs from more natural situations where n-3 fatty acids have a significant or even a predominant presence. This difference is largely accounted for by the diet. Whereas all the diets used under intensive conditions display by design an extremely heavy emphasis on linoleic acid to the virtual exclusion of any other polyunsaturates, natural situations supply a far more balanced polyunsaturated fatty acid spectrum. The often contested claim that the egg from a free range bird is of a better quality, more healthy and with a different taste may therefore not be without foundation. As can be seen from the Table 4, in terms of fatty acid content the egg of the alligator provides the most ideal mix. Unfortunately a range of factors preclude its ready availability, not least the hazard of egg collection!!

Present dietary attention is being very much directed to improving consumption of the specific omega-3 fatty acids, eicosapentaenoic and docosahexaenoic. The major natural sources of these fatty acids are oily fish, the consumption of which has been in singular decline over recent years and giving rise to major nutritional concerns. Following supplementation of these acids to the hen's diet, levels of 200-250 mg per egg have been achieved. This contrasts strongly with levels of only around 30 mg in eggs from hens fed standard diets. The level of omega-3s within a modified egg equates to more than fifty per cent of the advised daily requirement.

Increasing the egg level of long chain polyunsaturated fatty acids poses the question of possible problems of undesirable odour, arising from the fatty acid oxidation, especially as such acids are routinely supplied in the diet as fish oils or derivatives of fish oils. The problem however, can readily

Bizarre things that people do with eggs

The biggest scrambled egg

McDonald's achieved the amazing feat of setting a Guinness World Record in Christchurch, New Zealand when more than 20,000 free-range eggs were used to cook a scrambled egg, which weighed in at 1.24 tonnes.

The fastest omelette maker

Howard Helmer is the "World's Fastest Omelette Maker." A three-time record holder for his high-speed eggsperience, Howard holds the record as the fastest omelette cooker in the world by whipping up a whopping 427 omelettes in a mere 30 minutes. To earn his second and third world records, Howard flipped an omelette an amazing 30 times in 34 seconds before it broke and he cooked the fastest omelette ever recorded – 42 seconds from when the egg was cracked to when it was cooked.

be countered by appropriate addition of antioxidants. In the case of the egg, the possibility of any oxidation is well buffered naturally by a significant presence of the powerful anti-oxidant - vitamin E.

Where enhancement of n-3 fatty acid levels in the egg has been achieved through high levels of dietary fish oil incorporation, marked flavour effects have been reported. Some "off flavors" have also been observed when the dietary level of fish oil was significantly reduced. However, lipid derivatives of fish oils have achieved successful lipid manipulations without any taste effects, even up to the level of docosahexaenoic acid previously obtained from very high levels of fish oil inclusion.

Observations on polyunsaturated enriched eggs have shown no adverse effects on major production parameters, egg quality, aspects of culinary acceptability and molecular integrity of the polyunsaturates under the conditions of cooking.

A few studies exist that have evaluated potential physiological effects following consumption of the modified eggs. Some beneficial outcomes on plasma lipid profiles and blood pressure were observed following the consumption of eggs from hens fed a diet containing a substantial level of fish oil, but in view of the level of egg consumption (four eggs per day over a four week period) such data have to be viewed with some suspicion.

With requirements for long chain polyunsaturated of the n-3 series being maximal during the two extremes of life, namely foetal/neonatal development and ageing, specific areas of application have been suggested. Thus eggs with enhanced levels of docosahexaenoic acid could be used

Did you know that?

❖ The eggs we eat usually come from the chicken but it is quite common practice to eat eggs from other species of fowl, for example turkey, duck, goose, game birds, pigeon, quail, ostrich, pelican, a range of sea birds plus turtle, alligator, reptiles and even insect eggs. If it is egg shaped, then somebody somewhere will eat it!!

❖ The UK consumer preference is almost wholly for brown eggs. This is in contrast to some other European countries and the USA where the demand is for white eggs.

❖ Dirty eggs should never be washed in cold water. This causes the contents to shrink and allow bacterial invasion. Always use warm water for washing eggs.

❖ A simple way to tell if an egg is raw or has been cooked is to spin it. Lay the egg on a flat surface and spin gently. If it wobbles as it spins then it is raw.

during pregnancy and as a supplement to infant formulae and weaning diets. Similarly, in the elderly where the capacity to desaturate and chain-elongate alpha-linolenic acid to eicosapentaenoic and docosahexaenoic acids is severely reduced, the eggs may also have an important function to perform.

Suggestions for the dietary potential for omega-3 enriched eggs abound. However, it would be wise to remember that its purpose is solely as a simple and acceptable alternative delivery system for a valuable nutritional component. Titles such as the "Einstein" or "Harvard" egg, both of which have been used in commercial promotions, fail completely to keep the technology in perspective.

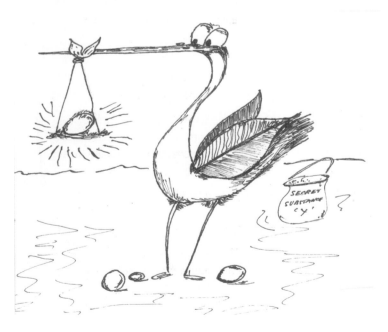

"For unto us a "super egg" is born and it shall be named…"

Vitamin A

Target tissue/functions:
forming and maintaining skeletal
and soft tissues, mucous membranes and
skin; promoting good vision and reproduction.

Deficiency symptoms: increased susceptibility to
infectious diseases; vision problems e.g. night
blindness; keratinisation of internal epithelia e.g. nasal
and respiratory passages.

Recommended Allowances:

EU RDA: 800 µg/day;
USA RDI: 700 - 1300 µg/day.

Vitamin D

Target tissue/Functions: regulation of absorption and body levels
of calcium and phosphorus and bone mineralization; aspects of body
growth and development; role in prevention of colon and rectal
cancer.

Deficiency symptoms: bone deformities e.g. rickets; bone
pain and muscle weakness.

Recommended Allowances:

EU RDA: 5 µg/day;
USA RDI: 15 - 20 µg/day.

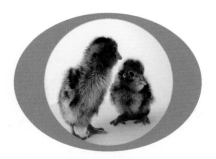

VITAMINS

The best vitamin for making friends - B1

Vitamins are dietary components essential for health and well-being. Initial recognition of this dates back to ancient Greece and dietary observation by Hypocrites, to be followed many centuries later by further similar connections between diet and health and ultimately culminating in the extensive "in depth" studies of the twentieth century.

The term vitamin very much reflects their history and function, being a combination of the word for life (vita) and major chemical features (the amines) of a vitamin.

The vitamin levels required in any diet to carry out their metabolic functions are very small indeed. Vitamins serve crucial functions in almost all body processes. In general their nutritional adequacy is served via the diet.

There are thirteen vitamins, divided and classified as being either water soluble (vitamin C and all the B complexes) or fat soluble (vitamins A, D, E and K). The solubility of the vitamin largely determines its function, mode of action, storage and toxicity.

Vitamin E

Target tissue/functions:
powerful anti-oxidative agent in protection of all body tissues and organs; promoting optimal development, growth, health.

Deficiency symptoms: fluid retention, anemia and lassitude; potential increased risk of heart and circulatory problems; premature ageing.

Recommended allowances:

EU RDA: 12 mg/day;
USA RDI: 15 - 19 mg/day.

Vitamin K

Target tissue/functions: blood clotting and erythrocyte function; bone health.

Deficiency symptoms: impaired blood clotting, bruising; extensive loss of blood; impaired tissue function.

Recommended allowances:

EU RDA: 75 µg/day;
USA RDI: 90 - 120 µg/day.

In contrast to the fat soluble vitamins, the water soluble vitamins exist only briefly within the body before transfer to the kidney and excretion via the urine. Their entry into the body from the diet is much freer than that of the fat soluble vitamins but once within the body, retention is far less. As a result, there is a far greater need for a consistent and regular pattern of intake for the water soluble vitamins to be effective.

Vitamin storage can give rise to an increase potential of toxicity. For instance, in the case of vitamins A and D where storage is wholly confined to the liver, toxicity arising from dietary overload can occur. In the absence of any significant storage of water-soluble vitamins, toxicity is confined to situations of prolonged periods of excessive intakes. Recommended dietary consumption of vitamins is highly influenced by features such as climate, age, basic health, pregnancy and lactation.

As can be seen from Table 5, eggs can be considered as a significant source of the recognised vitamins with one notable exception, namely vitamin C. All the B vitamins are present, plus the fat soluble vitamins A, D, E and K. Under normal dietary situations, significant levels of vitamins B2, B3, B5, B7, B9 and B12 are to be found.

In the case of vitamin B12, a single egg can deliver about forty four per cent of RDA. In view of the fact that this vitamin is in short supply within our daily diet, consumption of a single egg can perform a significant role in satisfying requirement. With the increasing awareness of the essentiality of vitamin B9 (folic acid) to our health and well being, in particular during pregnancy, its presence at seventeen per cent of RDA within the egg is also of significant importance.

Vitamin B1 (thiamine)

Target tissue/functions: tissue metabolism and health; nervous tissue function; promotion of energy metabolism.

Deficiency symptoms: fatigue, lassitude, depression, appetite loss, diminished mental function, muscle cramp, nausea, heart enlargement.

Recommended allowances:

EU RDA: 1.1 mg/day;
USA RDI: 1.1 - 1.4 mg/day

Vitamin B2 (riboflavin)

Target tissue/functions: general body/tissue growth and function; nerve and blood cell development; hormone regulation; tissue and mucus membrane repair; energy regulation.

Deficiency symptoms: fatigue; swollen and cracked mouth and tongue; anemia; depression; dry skin; potential promotion of cataracts.

Recommended allowances:

EU RDA: 1.4 mg/day;
USA RDI: 1.1 - 1.6 mg/day

Fat soluble vitamins can only be absorbed into the circulation from the intestine in conjunction with the fat components of the diet. As a result, any disease or disorder affecting fat absorption can potentially lead to a deficiency. Once within the circulation they are carried to the liver where, to a large extent they are also stored. The fat soluble vitamins are neither absorbed nor excreted from the body as readily as water soluble vitamins.

The unique and special metabolic roles of vitamins E and K highlight their potential dietary importance within the egg. Vitamin E in particular has a significant nutritional role to play through its function as an important part of the complex antioxidant systems that are required to maintain the chemical and functional stability of major metabolic systems within our body. The nutritional significance of vitamin K is its important role in circulatory stability.

Although a vast amount is now known about individual functions and requirements for the vitamins within our diet, modern research is still coming up with new findings and significant surprises. For instance, the term vitamin D is most well known as a constituent within cod liver oil that cures rickets and plays a critically important role in the development, growth and mineralisation of the skeleton, in particular during the formative years but also throughout life. In its active hormonal form it is required for a balanced intestinal absorption and subsequent distribution of calcium.

It has become regularly referred to as "sunshine vitamin" almost solely for its function for bone health. However, new data has revealed that vitamin D plays some very important roles far beyond bone formation and maintenance. Current research is now documenting a significant number of diseases and conditions in which an insufficient vitamin D intake is

Vitamin
B3 (niacin)

Target tissue/functions: specific enzymes for promotion of cell metabolism; hormone synthesis, skin and nervous tissue function; regulation of blood lipid levels; nutrient assimilation.

Deficiency symptoms: dermatitis; sore mouth; loss of appetite, digestive upsets; anxiety complex; depression; dementia.

Recommended allowances:

EU RDA: 16 mg/day;
USA RDI: 14 - 18 mg/day.

Vitamin B5 (pantothenic acid)

Target tissue/functions: co-enzyme in nutrient assimilation and metabolism; promotion of growth and development.

Deficiency symptoms: excessive fatigue; sleep deprivation; loss of appetite, nausea; dermatitis.

Recommended allowances:

EU RDA: 6 mg/day;
USA RDI: 5 - 7 mg/day

clearly involved, the list including several common cancers, diabetes, rheumatoid arthritis and multiple sclerosis. An activated form of vitamin D has now been identified that can help in stabilising blood pressure, suppressing artery-damaging inflammation and protect blood vessels from calcification together with a role in the modulation of immune function and thereby inflammatory response.

Table 5. Vitamin supply from a large (60g) egg

Vitamin	Content in egg	% RDA
A, µg	150	18.8
D, µg	1.5	30.0
E, mg	1.1	9.2
K, µg	25.0	33.3
B1, µg	50.0	4.6
B2, µg	160	11.4
B3, mg	1.6	10.0
B5, µg	850	14.2
B6, µg	60.0	4.3
B7, µg	13.3	26.6
B9, µg	34.0	17.0
B12, µg	1.1	44.0

Vitamin B6 (pyridoxine)

Target tissue/functions: co-enzyme in nutrient assimilation and metabolism; formation of red blood cells; brain function; antibody synthesis; nerve function.

Deficiency symptoms: weakness; mental confusion; irritability; sleep deprivation; hyperactivity; anemia; skin lesions; kidney stones.

Recommended allowances:
EU RDA: 1.4 mg/day;
USA RDI: 1.3 - 2.0 mg/day.

Vitamin B7 (biotin)

Target tissue/functions: nutrient assimilation and metabolism; hormone and cholesterol synthesis; overall development and health.

Deficiency symptoms: hair loss; facial and genital rash; depression; lethargy; hallucinations; numbness and tingling in extremities; muscle pain; loss of appetite; reduced immunity.

Recommended allowances:
EU RDA: 50 µg/day ;
USA RDI: 30 - 35 µg/day.

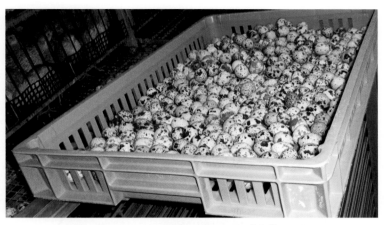

Quail eggs are not just for a cocktail party

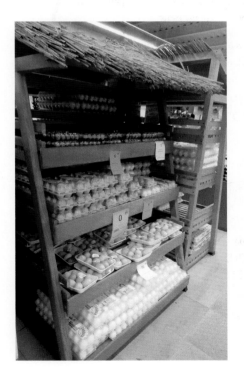

Egg presentation in the shop can be quite creative

Vitamin B9 (folic acid)

Target tissue/functions: red blood cell formation; synthesis of DNA; foetal development; cardiovascular health; cognitive and nerve function; nutrient uptake.

Deficiency symptoms: anemia; mood swings; gastro-intestinal disorders; foetal neural defects during pregnancy.

Recommended allowances:
EU RDA: 200 µg/day;
USA RDI: 400 - 600 µg/day

Vitamin B12

Target tissue/functions: coenzyme for DNA synthesis; promotion of cell development and metabolism; formation, growth and division of red blood cells; haemoglobin synthesis; nerve function.

Deficiency symptoms: numbness in limbs; walking difficulties; memory loss; disorientation; dementia; loss of appetite; digestive upsets; nausea; depression.

Recommended allowances:
EU RDA: 2.5 µg/day;
USA RDI: 2.4 - 2.8 µg/day

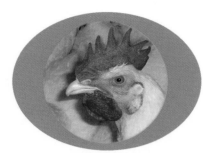

MINERALS

Strike while the iron's hot

Minerals are present throughout the body. Something of the order of sixty different minerals exist within the body of which twenty two can be considered to be significantly important to human health and welfare. However, it has been speculated that at some time in the future all the chemical elements will be recognised as having a biological role to play.

Distribution of the mineral elements varies considerably depending upon the tissue and its function. Those present at significant levels are referred to as major elements, for example the presence of calcium in the bone. Those present only in minute quantities are referred to as trace elements which, in some instances, have a quantitative presence that is virtually undetectable. The level of any element is no guide to its functional importance.

Elemental roles range from structural involvements in tissue and cells to intimate metabolic actions that are essential for health, reproduction and life itself. The major function of trace elements is their requirement as activators for metabolism - for example, enzyme reactions, components to

Calcium

Target tissue/functions:
skeletal structure; teeth; blood clotting; enzyme function; cell fluid balance; heart action; muscle contraction; nerve action.

Deficiency symptoms: fragile bone and tooth structure; retarded growth; osteoporosis; insomnia; irritability; muscle sensitivity.

Recommended allowances:

EU RDA: 800 mg/day;
USA RDI: 1000 - 1300 mg/day.

Phosphorus

Target tissue/functions: skeletal structure; teeth; nutritional uptake and metabolism; balance of cell and blood composition; nerve tissues; brain cells.

Deficiency symptoms: hardly ever detectable but effects on bone structure, general growth, nerve and brain function and general lassitude.

Recommended allowances:

EU RDA: 700 mg/day;
USA RDI: 700 - 1250 mg/day

aid the passage of macro- and micro-nutrients between cells and body fluids, oxygen transport and exchange, control of acidity/alkalinity and nerve transmission. Although some mineral functions can be achieved alone, in the majority of cases they are achieved by attachment to other chemical components, for example proteins.

The following ten minerals found in eggs in substantial quantities are of particular significance to tissue function and health. It is necessary to underline that as in the case of vitamins, mineral requirements and therefore RDA's and RDI's, can be highly influenced by a range of features, such as climate, age, basic health, pregnancy and lactation and other features.

As can be seen from Table 6, in overall terms the mineral content of the egg makes a significant contribution across the board to human requirements. Although all are of nutritional importance, of particular note with respect to RDA and RDI requirements are the contributions by the egg of iodine and selenium whose functional involvements in metabolism are increasingly being realised.

Iodine is the essential requirement for a fully functional thyroid gland which is a major key to the hormonal regulation of a wide and notable range of metabolic functions. In historic terms, the importance of selenium to health and well-being is, to say the least, highly controversial. There exists a very fine line delineating the element's toxicity and its essentiality in the diet. Indeed, until the early 1970's interest in the element was solely confined to its existence as the cause of a selection of very debilitating diseases and conditions prevalent in various parts of the world associated with plants displaying a high content of selenium.

Potassium

Target tissue/functions:
acid-alkaline balance in blood and
tissues; muscle contraction; blood/kidney
detoxification; tissue healing and elasticity;
heart rhythm; intracellular fluid balance.

Deficiency symptoms: liver ailments; impaired
healing; reduced muscle control and fatigue; digestive
upsets; edema; high blood pressure and increased potential
of cardiac impairment.

Recommended allowances:
EU RDA: 2 g/day;
USA RDI: 4.7 - 5.1 g/day.

Sodium

Target tissue/functions: whole body fluid balance; elimination of
carbon dioxide; muscle and nerve function; iron uptake.

Deficiency symptoms: muscle weakness; exhaustion; apathy;
nausea; gall bladder and kidney stones; muscle cramp.

Recommended allowances:
EU RDA: 0.5 - 3.5 g/day;
USA RDI: 1.2 - 1.5 g/day.

The association of selenium with important aspects of our metabolism is therefore a recent phenomenon. It is based on an initial recognition of a dependency for the element within an important array of tissue enzymes and the suggestion of a potential role in the prevention of certain cancers.

It has now been established that there are at least twenty five selenoproteins, i.e. enzymes containing selenium in their active centres, required for the regulation of important biochemical processes in the body. This function is mainly operated through the major roles the enzymes play, in conjunction with fellow minor elements such as copper and zinc, in the detoxification of peroxides and free radicals. Peroxides and free radicals are natural products of metabolism and, if not controlled, are responsible for extensive functional damage.

The manifestations of an inadequate selenium consumption are extensive, involving a wide range of pathological, physiological and metabolic problems. They include enhanced skin and scalp conditions, growth retardation, muscular pain and a general lassitude, reduced defence against bacterial and viral infections and, more dramatically, decreased male and female fertility. Selenium deficiency is now recognised as a global problem in urgent need of a rectification.

With direct dietary supplementation being seen as the easiest means of enhancing selenium supply, considerable attention has and continues to be paid to the egg as a means of supplemental delivery. The egg's position as a traditional and affordable food in almost all countries, and its consumption by people of all ages on a regular basis, is seen as a possible safe vehicle for selenium supplementation.

Copper

Target tissue/functions: catalyst for many biochemical processes; absorption and metabolism of iron; red blood cell, connective tissues and nerve structure formation; skin pigmentation.

Deficiency symptoms: as for iron e.g. retarded haemoglobin production; general debility; reduced growth etc.

Recommended allowances:
EU RDA: 1 mg/day;
USA RDI: 0.9 - 1.3 mg/day

Iodine

Target tissue/functions: the thyroid gland for thyroxine formation for regulation of bodily metabolism; oxidation of fats and proteins; circulatory balance.

Deficiency symptoms: enlargement of thyroid gland (goitre); cretinism (subnormal metabolism); low physical and mental activity; nerve dysfunction; mental retardation in infants.

Recommended allowances:
EU RDA: 0.15 mg;
USA RDI: 0.15 - 0.29 mg/day.

Table 6. Mineral supply from a large (60 g) egg

Mineral	Content in egg	% RDA
Sodium, mg	69.2	4.6
Potassium, mg	78.7	3.9
Calcium, mg	28.0	3.5
Phosphorus, mg	96.5	13.8
Magnesium, mg	5.9	1.6
Iron, mg	1.1	7.9
Iodine, µg	16.9	11.3
Copper, mg	0.075	7.5
Zinc, mg	0.75	7.5
Selenium, µg	12.5	22.7

Zinc

Target tissue/functions: wound healing; insulin manufacture and therefore blood sugar regulation; growth and reproduction; the immune system; sense of smell and taste.

Deficiency symptoms: prostate trouble; depression; absence of taste and smell; defective intestinal absorption; growth restriction.

Recommended allowances:

EU RDA: 10 mg/day;
USA RDI: 8 - 13 mg/day.

Selenium

Target tissue/functions: integral part of selenoproteins, essential for a wide range of metabolic functions e.g. antioxidant defence system, immunity, thyroid action.

Deficiency symptoms: severely reduced immune-competence; increased sensitivity to disease and infection, including cancers.

Recommended allowances:

EU RDA: 55 μg/day;
USA RDI: 55 - 70

To this end, selenium enriched eggs each containing some 30-35 µg of selenium per egg and therefore able to satisfy some fifty per cent of RDA, are available in more than twenty five countries of the world, albeit at present mainly concentrated in Eastern Europe and the Far East.

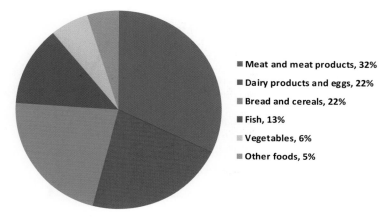

■ Meat and meat products, 32%

■ Dairy products and eggs, 22%

■ Bread and cereals, 22%

■ Fish, 13%

■ Vegetables, 6%

■ Other foods, 5%

Estimated intake of Se from different components of the UK diet

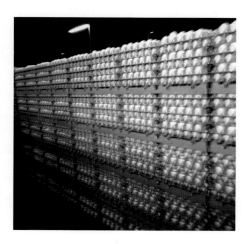

Commercial egg storage is always a challenge

Magnesium

Target tissue/functions:
participation in more than 300
enzyme reactions in the body; protein
formation and cell replication; nerve and
muscle tissue formation.

Deficiency symptoms: nervousness and irritability;
accelerated heartbeat; digestive disorders; soft bones;
increased excretion of calcium; fatigue; mental confusion;
weakness and muscle cramps; loss of appetite.

Recommended allowances:
EU RDA: 375 mg/day;
USA RDI: 310 - 420 mg/day.

Iron

Target tissue/functions: haemoglobin synthesis and red blood cell
quality; bone marrow, liver and spleen metabolism; growth and
energy production.

Deficiency symptoms: anaemia; brittle hair; digestive
disturbances; fatigue; dizziness; fragile bones; slowed mental
reactions; nervousness; ridging of nails.

Recommended allowances:
EU RDA: 14 mg/day;
USA RDI: 8 - 27 mg/day.

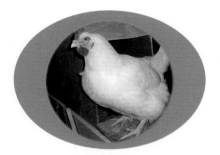

CHOLINE

"a belated recognition"

Our diet and its nutritional components can readily be divided into two camps. There are the "foot soldiers" which make up the bulk of everything we eat. These are the unsung heroes whose major function is to supply our basic needs in terms of energy and tissue regeneration so essential to survival and, at the same time, satisfying our appetites and nutritional bulk requirements. Such are exemplified by overall groupings such the carbohydrates, proteins etc.

Then there are what might best be referred to as the dietary "prima donnas" whose intake at notably lower or even minute levels are required for highly specific metabolic functions and whose actions far outweigh their absolute presence. These are most notably represented by the vitamins and minerals.

However, somewhere between these two groups, metabolites exist that perform a dual role. Their primary function is as adjuncts to the metabolic role of large molecular complexes. Following release from such roles they then take on for themselves a range of essential functions in specific aspects of metabolism.

**Table 7. Choline provision
in selected food items**

Food	Serving, g	Choline, mg
Salmon	80	198
Chicken egg	60	133
Chicken	80	59
Sausage	80	58
Milk	212	40
Cauliflower	60	25
Peas	60	23
Almonds	27	16
Broccoli	60	21

Examples of this would be the relationship that exists between dietary protein supply and its subsequent breakdown into its essential and non essential amino acids; similarly the release of essential and non essential fatty acids from lipids. These are obvious and major examples. There also exists a range of less obvious examples of this duplicitous role in form and function. The presence of the metabolite choline within the egg is one such example.

It took more than one hundred years from the discovery of choline to its recognition as an important nutrient. Indeed, choline was discovered in 1862 and chemically synthesised some four years later. Following the observation in 1946 that a choline-deficient diet led to liver cancer in rats, and the discovery just a few years later that it was an essential for nerve function, choline became officially recognised as an essential nutrient in 1998. A remarkably lengthy gestation period between discovery and dietary recognition!

The importance of choline in a wide range of critical metabolic functions is now well established. Apart from its role in maintaining a balanced liver function, choline plays a critical role in brain development, neurotransmissions, memory and elements of cognition. There is a particular requirement during foetal development and the immediate post natal period. A reduced choline intake is also now implicated in blood compositional changes associated with an increased risk of several chronic conditions that include specific cancers.

Choline is a major component within the phospholipids. Phospholipids are the second major lipid fraction within the egg yolk accounting for some twenty five percent of total lipid content. In absolute terms, a 60 gram egg contains

Bizarre things that people do with eggs

The largest omelette

On the 8th October 2010 the world's largest omelette was created in Turkey. To achieve the record feat, an enthusiastic team of 10 chefs and 50 cooks was formed. The record to beat was an omelette weighing 3.625 tonnes set in South Africa in 2009.

Compliance with guidance for Guinness World Records was essential for the successful outcome of the attempt. The finished omelette had to be edible, include eggs and oil or butter and be a scaled-up version of a normal omelette. After the official tare weigh-in, 110,000 pasteurised organic liquid eggs, supplied in a large refrigerated truck just before the start of the event, were poured into the pan along with 300 litres of oil and salt. The chefs and cooks kept a careful eye on the omelette for over two hours, indefatigably stirring it to mix the ingredients and to ensure it was evenly cooked.

The ultimate weight was a staggering 4.401 tonnes, thereby establishing the attempt as a new Guinness World Record achievement. At the announcement, a deafening cheer erupted and the celebrations began with enthusiastic omelette tasting.

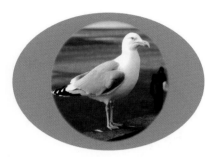

CAROTENE AND CAROTENOIDS

"........seeing is believing........."

U nder natural circumstances the diet of the hen includes a significant proportion of vegetable material, thereby enabling a wider range of dietary components to be incorporated into the egg compared to the commercial hen. A feature of most plants and vegetables is a presence of highly pigmented components and accordingly free-range eggs routinely display significantly pigmented yolks.

As a result of comparison with the pallid appearance of intensively produced eggs, but based on no scientific evidence, the consumer arbitrarily correlates this as being indicative of an enhanced healthiness.

However, to assuage this consumer preference, it is now a routine part of intensive production systems to imbue all eggs with the desired "healthy" glow by means of precise incorporation of plant pigments into the hen's basic diet. Although this was originally viewed solely as a cosmetic indulgence, it is now being increasingly recognised that the presence of the plant pigments in the egg does indeed have a positive health benefit.

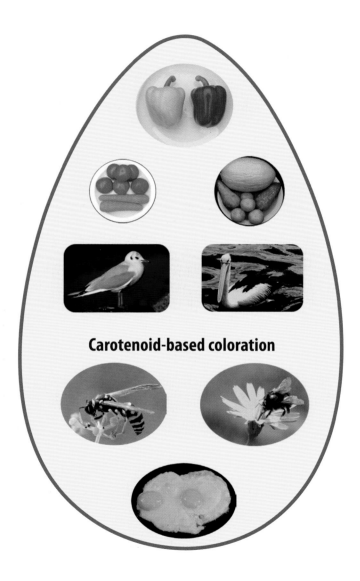

Carotenoid-based coloration

Simplistically, the plant pigments come under the single title of "carotene". In reality this encompasses more than seven hundred components, the carotenoids, of which only a proportion are consumed in the diet. Until recently any nutritional role for the carotenoids was seen as being confined to that of a precursor for vitamin A. Now, however, there is accumulating evidence of a significant role on their own account in aspects of health promotion. Animal studies have demonstrated a positive regression in certain cancer tumours during conditions of enhanced intakes of carotenoids.

Carotenoids possess powerful antioxidant capacities. They may therefore play a significant part in the prevention of destructive oxidation processes that are an ever significant but natural part of our metabolism. Presently there is particular interest in the positive part the carotenoids may play in the maintenance of visual health and the prevention of the age related degenerative condition known as macular degeneration. This is an increasingly common condition of the ageing process and is manifested by an impairment of central vision through the destruction of retinal photo-reception. Much contemporary interest is devoted to the potential beneficial role that can be played in this condition by two specific carotenoids, lutein and zeaxanthin, through their proven ability to reduce photo-oxidation within the retina.

Increasing the levels of both lutein and zeaxanthin in the hen's diet readily gives rise to their enhancement within the egg yolk. Consumption of such enhanced eggs at a rate of one or two per day increases blood plasma levels of both compounds by between fifty and one hundred percent above normal and resulting in significant positive effects upon their concentrations within the retina.

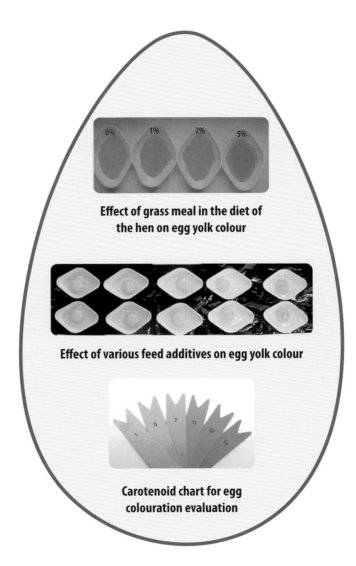

**Effect of grass meal in the diet of
the hen on egg yolk colour**

Effect of various feed additives on egg yolk colour

**Carotenoid chart for egg
colouration evaluation**

Both lutein and zeaxanthin are fat soluble compounds and therefore are most efficiently absorbed from the diet in the presence of a fatty environment. In this respect therefore, their delivery via the yolk may also serve to promote their intestinal uptake.

The promotion of lutein and zeaxanthin levels in the egg can be problematical as due attention has to be paid to the significant compositional variation of diets in the modern egg production systems. However, since it is possible to compose a supplemental package of the two carotenoids for inclusion into any diet, this should really present no real problem. Data obtained to date would most certainly indicate the undoubted potential of plant carotenoids in further enhancing the egg's portfolio of wholesome and healthy components.

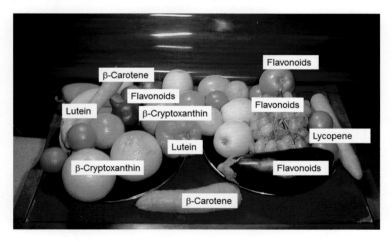

Fruit and vegetables are good sources of carotenoids

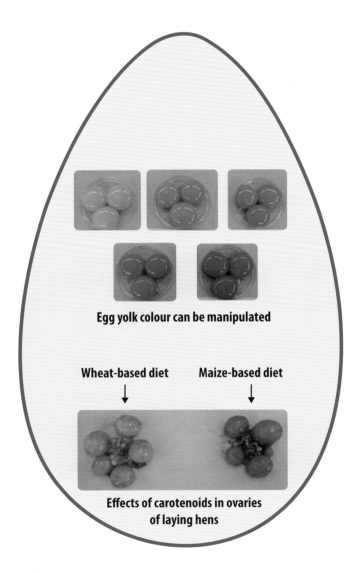

Egg yolk colour can be manipulated

Wheat-based diet   **Maize-based diet**

**Effects of carotenoids in ovaries
of laying hens**

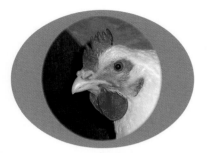

ANTIOXIDANTS AND HUMAN HEALTH

Diet cures more than the lancet

Survival on earth, whether it be animals, plants or micro-organisms, would be impossible without oxygen. However, over recent years research has increasingly become focused on the adverse metabolic effects of oxygen to our lives. These arise from compounds containing what are referred to as activated molecules of oxygen or more commonly known as "free radicals". They can damage various biological molecules and disrupt their metabolism.

The presence of free radicals, either at high or low concentrations, is a price that has to be paid in return for the "pleasure and privilege" derived from living in an oxygenated environment. The benefits that oxygen gives to us all on the one hand is, to a greater or lesser extent, taken away on the other hand through its ability to be metabolically transformed into highly tissue-destructive free radicals.

Free radicals are constantly being formed as a natural consequence of the body's metabolism. With all cells in the body continuously producing free radicals, their overall synthesis under normal circumstances is truly enormous. An annual

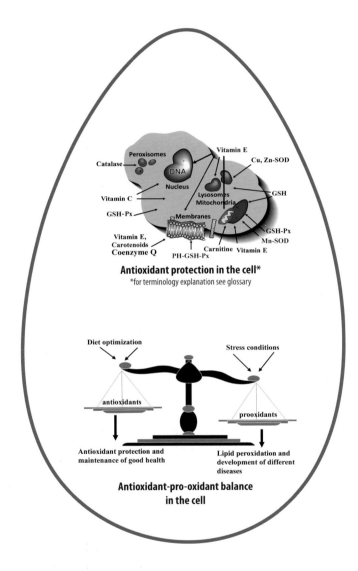

Antioxidant protection in the cell*
*for terminology explanation see glossary

Antioxidant-pro-oxidant balance in the cell

production rate has been calculated as some 1.72kg. Certain aspects of modern life are extremely adept at increasing this production even further - smoking being the most potent. The enormity of free radical output and its toxic properties is such that the body has necessarily had to devise a range of antioxidant systems that enable cell protection and therefore maintain the metabolic balance essential for survival.

Paramount in the role of antioxidant protection are two main players - vitamin E and the mineral element selenium. As vitamin E cannot be synthesised in the body, an adequate intake is reliant upon adherence to a well balanced diet, but taking into account the fact that vitamin E suffers from some inherent instability.

Vitamin E is recognised as the main biological antioxidant and thus plays a key role in antioxidant defence. As a result, enhancement of vitamin E intake helps to ensure adequate antioxidant protection and thus appropriate benefits to all aspects of our health. In general, uptake of extra vitamin E is best assured from natural dietary components in preference to artificial supplementation.

As already stated, there exists a very fine line that delineates the essentiality of selenium and its toxicity. Its essentiality is based on functional requirement to a raft of tissue enzymes whose actions are major contributors in the detoxification of peroxides and free radicals. With direct dietary supplementation being seen as an easy and reliable means of both vitamin E and selenium deliveries, some considerable attention is being paid to the egg as a convenient means of delivery.

The egg's position as a traditional and affordable food in almost all countries of the world, and its consumption by

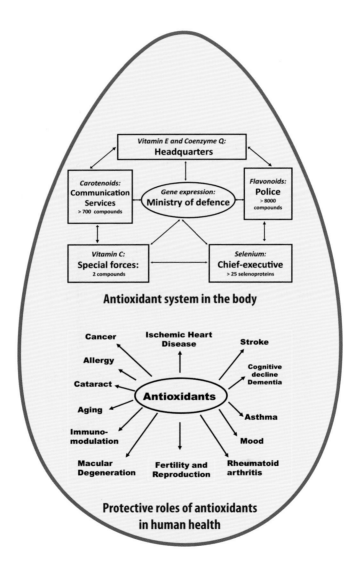

Antioxidant system in the body

Protective roles of antioxidants in human health

all age groups, makes it a reliable and easy vehicle for supplemental delivery of a range of dietary metabolites and not least for delivery of vitamin E and selenium.

With vitamin E levels in the egg being closely dependent upon its level in the hen's diet, the technology for a production of vitamin E-enriched eggs has been developed. It is now possible to tailor a single egg able to deliver a full daily requirement of vitamin E. In the case of selenium, fortified eggs are freely available under a plethora of names and brands in more than twenty five countries, the major production sites being in Eastern Europe and the Far East. The most common level of selenium delivery per egg is 30 - 35µg which is sufficient to satisfy some fifty per cent of our daily dietary requirement.

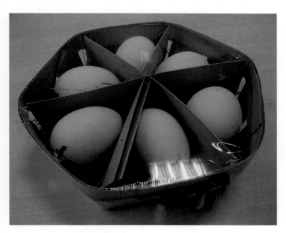

Table 8. Natural food sources of some antioxidants

Vitamin E	Oilseeds, vegetable oils, nuts, whole grains, cereals, margarine, etc.
Vitamin C	Fruits and vegetables, berries, citrus fruits, etc.
Carotenoids	Dark leafy vegetables, carrots, sweet potatoes, tomatoes, apricots, citrus fruits, kale, etc.
Flavonoids/isoflavonoids	Fruits and vegetables, oil-seeds, berries, peppers, citrus fruits, tomatoes, onions, etc.
Phenolic acids	Oilseeds, cereals, grains, etc.
Catechins	Green tea, berries, certain oilseeds, etc.
Extracts/essential oils	Green tea, rosemary, sage, clove, oregano, thyme, oat, rice bran, etc.

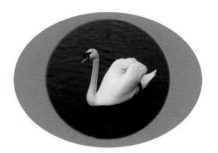

SATIETY AND WEIGHT LOSS

He who eats when he is full digs his grave with his teeth

The prevalence of excess body weight is seen as one of the biggest health issues of contemporary society affecting all ages and social classes. In spite of efforts at all levels (governmental, scientific etc.,) to underline the dangers arising from being overweight, the public remains steadfastly immune to the adoption of any lifestyle that might reverse or even slow down the advance of weight gain and obesity.

The message that weight loss in the main comes down to calorie intake is well known, but unfortunately this is countered by the surfeit and variety of food available and our insatiable desire to consume it. Under these conditions can the egg play any positive part in making some change, however small, to weight loss? The current immediate answer in this "David versus Goliath" encounter would be appear to be "no".

However, in light of what is now known about the egg's chemistry there exist certain features that alone may be helpful, the more-so in the presence of other dietary

EGG COCKTAILS

Eggs are an important part of many classical cocktails, providing unmatched texture and mouth feel. Some of the best known cocktails that use eggs are eggnog, flips and sours.

Eggnog (or egg nog) is a sweetened dairy-based beverage traditionally made with milk and/or cream, sugar, beaten eggs and liquor. Brandy, rum, moonshine, or whisky is sometimes added and the finished serving may be garnished with a sprinkling of ground cinnamon or nutmeg.

A flip is a similar class of mixed drinks, containing egg, alcoholic drink (whiskey, cognac, port, bourbon, etc) and sugar.

Sours are mixed drinks containing a base liquor (bourbon or some other whiskey in the case of a whiskey sour), lemon or lime juice, egg white, and a sweetener (triple sec, simple syrup, grenadine, or pineapple juice are common).

adjuncts. It is well known that increased protein intake is a better positive mediating influence on satiation than other major components of the diet. The egg has a high protein content which, in combination with its low energy density, provides a satisfying effect on appetite whilst at the same time maintaining a low calorie intake (one egg provides 6 grams of protein at a cost of only 75 calories).

An important finding from recent research into aspects of dietary control has been the isolation from the stomach of a hitherto unknown hormone, ghrelin, whose primary function includes the switching on/off a desire to eat. Ghrelin has been shown to be released in a time-dependant manner, appropriately increasing before meals and decreasing after meals. Interestingly, foods with high protein levels such as eggs reduce ghrelin secretion, thereby promoting a feeling of satiation. A selection of controlled clinical experiments has been conducted on the effects of egg intake on satiation. All have involved overweight and obese participants.

Outcomes for the trials were all similar, namely that eating a diet based on eggs induced greater satiety, reduced perceived cravings and gave rise to less desire to eat over a subsequent period. For example, an induced feeling of fullness following breakfast resulted in a reduced desire to eat at the next meal which in several cases was observed to extend as far as twenty four hours later.

There is no doubt that such findings suggest that a regular inclusion of eggs in the diet may be of positive benefit in situations requiring weight loss or, at least the maintenance of weight stability.

A selection of egg based diets has been devised with notable claims of weight loss and reduced appetite. Most notably,

EGG LIQUORS

There is a range of egg-containing liquors with Advocaat being most well known. Advocaat (or advokat) is a rich and creamy liqueur made from eggs, sugar and brandy. It has a smooth, custard-like flavour. The exact recipe was invented by the corporate founder Eugen Verpoorten 1876 and has now been with the Verpoortens for five generations and its exact composition is a corporate secret. Up to 1.3 million fresh Class A eggs are used daily in production.

Originally, Advocaat was an avocado liquor made by Dutch traders in South America. When they got home, avocados were unavailable but eggs made a similarly textured beverage. It is also a versatile culinary item that can be used in preparing soups, cakes, steak, fish, and many other dishes.

The German equivalent is called Eierlikör (literally "egg liqueur"). It is based on either brandy or rectified spirit. The Polish equivalent called ajerkoniak is based on vodka instead of brandy, despite what the name may suggest. Rompope of Puebla, Mexico, and Sabajón of Colombia are very similar liquors based on egg yolk and vanilla. Some varieties have additional flavourings.

published personal papers of ex-Prime Minister Thatcher record a positive weight loss that resulted from a period on such a diet which included a consumption of twenty eight eggs per week.

Of a more extreme quotable example is that of the art collector Charles Saatchi who, over a period of some ten months of eating eggs at the rate of nine per day, achieved a weight loss of sixty pounds. Sadly, in both cases the effects on other aspects resulting from such high daily consumption of eggs are left to our imagination!

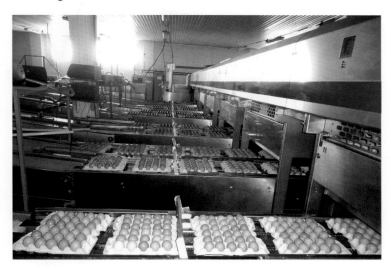

Eggs are sorted out automatically

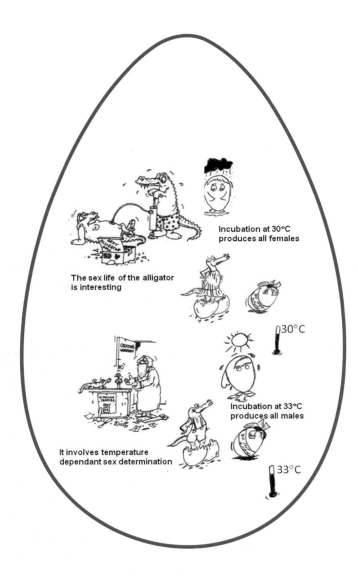

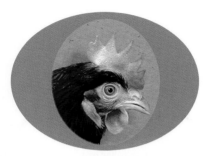

THE EGG - A POSITIVE ROLE IN EXERCISE

Prevention is better than cure

Diet and exercise go hand in glove. This may be seen as of particular importance to athletes where there is an ultimate requirement to maintain muscle tissue and function. Under these circumstances, extreme attention has to be paid to both nutritional adequacy and quality.

For lesser mortals attempting to maintain a degree of fitness and activity required for a healthy lifestyle, nutrient adequacy and quality are of no less importance. As in the case of the athlete, it has long been recognised that where there is regular indulgence in any physical activity, then it is most important that adequate attention be paid to dietary protein levels to satisfy muscle growth and repair.

Data on the daily protein requirement to sustain basic health and cellular function has been estimated at around 0.3 grams per pound of body weight, the requirement increasing some three-fold under conditions of severe exercise as undertaken by athletes. Such data are not absolute due to differences in body structure, the nature of the exercise and protein quality.

Eggs as art

Russian Tsar Nicholas II used to
commission jewelled eggs as Christmas
gifts for members of Russia's royal family.
Some of these made by jeweller Carl Faberge, are
now collector's items worth millions of dollars; Carl
Faberge created the world's most valuable eggs for the
Russian ruler Tsar Alexander III as a present for his wife.
They are made of gold and decorated with jewels. Inside one
of the eggs was a tiny hen with ruby eyes. The most expensive
egg ever sold was the Faberge "Winter egg" costing 5.5 million
US dollars in 1994.

The history of decorating eggs goes back to ancient times. All
cultures have, at one time or another, had a tradition of decorating
and giving eggs as gifts.

Goose, duck and hens' eggs are usually "blown" - a hole is made in
either end and the contents are blown out. The egg is then
exquisitely decorated by carving, dyeing and painting, using a
number of different techniques.

Many of those early techniques and traditions are
continued today by folk artists around the world.

The best proteins are recognised as those derived from animal sources. In particular, the egg is recognised as occupying the prime position through its high quality amino acid profile, high nitrogen utilisation rating and ease of digestion. Intake of egg protein in both powder and liquid formats is widely undertaken by athletes.

However, in modern times and to accommodate contemporary tastes, egg protein itself is now more often obtained through the consumption of the whole egg via the standard and substantial range of culinary offerings. As a result, there is a further contribution of high quality protein delivered by the yolk accompanied also by an important admixture of essential vitamins, minerals and lipid metabolites. For instance, arachidonic acid which is a significant component of the yolk lipid, is the principle building block in the production of metabolites known as prostaglandins which are proven to have a selection of roles in both muscle stimulation and growth. In athletics involving acts of high physical loading e.g. weight lifting, enhanced egg consumption is seen as a dietary essential.

Egg consumption is therefore now increasingly being recognised to have a beneficial input not only for athletes but also for the ordinary person who takes regular exercise as part of their lifestyle.

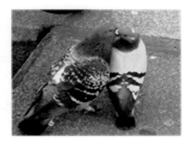

Bizarre things that people do with eggs

The most eggs eaten by a person

Sixty five hard boiled eggs were eaten in 6 minutes and 40 seconds by Sonya Thomas from Alexandria, USA. She was 43 years old and her weight was 105 kg.

The most eggs held in the hand

The record for the most eggs held in the hand is seventeen and was achieved by Rob Beaton in Ocean Gate, New Jersey, USA, on the 10th January 2007.

The largest number of eggs cracked in an hour

Bob Blumer, host of "Glutton for Punishment" on the Food Network, has set the World Record for the most number of eggs cracked in an hour. How many eggs would you have to crack to beat his record? A mere 2,071! And you'd have to crack those eggs using just one hand! In fact, Blumer actually cracked 2,318 eggs, but there was broken eggshell in 248 of those eggs and they were discounted.

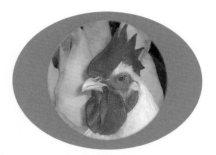

NUTRITIONAL ENHANCEMENT OF EGGS

An egg today is better than a hen tomorrow

As in most instances concerning animal tissues and their metabolism, the nutrient composition of the egg is very much open to change through the diet. Corn and soya are routinely the main ingredients in countries where their supply is cheap and plentiful e.g. the United States and Canada. In European countries where corn and soya are relatively expensive, the diet has to be significantly supplemented with grains such as wheat and barley. To meet the necessary requirements of the commercial hen for vitamins, minerals and certain amino acids, the diet is further supplemented with a specifically prepared "premix" to meet any shortfalls.

In general terms, the egg displays a remarkably stable nutritional composition in line with its original function, namely that of satisfying the necessary requirements for embryo development and healthy chick emergence. Where circumstances require, then changes can be forced upon egg composition. Such is the case in modern egg production systems. Required egg outputs in commercial practice would never be achieved without intervention into aspects of the hen's feed.

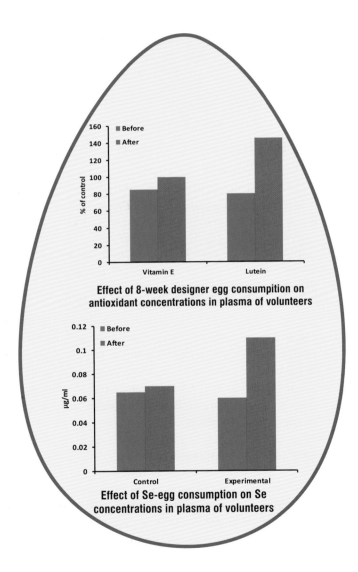

Effect of 8-week designer egg consumpition on antioxidant concentrations in plasma of volunteers

Effect of Se-egg consumption on Se concentrations in plasma of volunteers

As has already been fully discussed, the basic egg deserves recognition for its ability to supply a high quality regimen of nutritional components to our diet. However, the opportunity is now seen for the egg to play an even greater dietary role to that ever previously expected by using the egg as a delivery system.

A constant flow of information on dietary essentials, in combination with technical abilities to manipulate the egg's nutritional content and, last but not least, the increasing awareness of widespread health problems within society, has prompted the concept of so called "designer" or "nutritionally enhanced" eggs. Although the potential exists for enhancement of almost any metabolite in the egg, those presently seen of major commercial interest are the omega-3 series of unsaturated fatty acids, vitamin E, carotenoids and selenium whose nutritional values have already been described.

The idea of a designer egg may be considered to some extent as merely going back to nature. The major driving force of intensive commercialisation is supply and unit costs. Praiseworthy as it has been, it has not been achieved without some shortcomings to the egg's nutritional quality. As has been highlighted, it is now widely realised that there are some notable quality differences between eggs of wild species and birds kept under more natural conditions compared to intensively maintained birds.

Indeed, it may be said that nature has been once more proved to be right. Those essential nutrients displaying an obvious reduction in the commercial egg are also those that play a significant role in embryo development and chick survival; also, in turn, for our health.

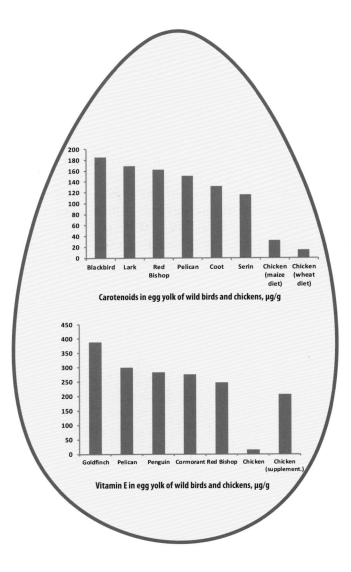

Carotenoids in egg yolk of wild birds and chickens, µg/g

Vitamin E in egg yolk of wild birds and chickens, µg/g

Therefore the initial choices for nutritional fortification of the egg are of no surprise. It is nothing other than returning egg composition back to something like its natural state with the added potential of being able to take matters even further.

In general the poultry industry has not been quick to accept and apply such technology and where it has, most notably in East European countries and Russia, it only accounts for some 5-10 per cent of total egg sales. However, there are examples (in Ukraine, for example) where nutritionally enhanced egg production has moved from the niche market to the main stream.

Clearly, nutritional fortification of the egg does not come without an additional cost above that of the conventional egg. However, where enhancement of the egg with vitamin E, carotenoids and selenium has been undertaken the cost of production of a fortified egg has remained comparable to that of its free-range counterpart.

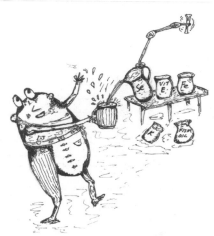

Egg-cellent stuff

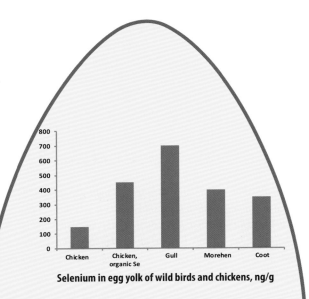

Selenium in egg yolk of wild birds and chickens, ng/g

Table 9. Possibilities of egg enrichment with antioxidants

Antioxidant	Egg enrichment
Vitamin E	Yes
Selenium	Yes
Carotenoids	Yes
Vitamin C	No
Flavonoids	No
Essential oils	No
Glutathione	No

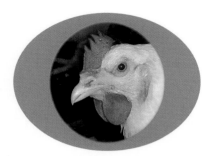

EGG PRESERVATION - FROM ANCIENT TIMES TO THE PRESENT

Don't put all your eggs in one basket

Need to store some eggs? Simple - put them in the fridge where they will keep for several weeks or even a month or two. But what of the past when fridges did not exist or were not available. Eggs have always been seen as a commodity which requires to be "on tap". Egg preservation has a very ancient and successful history tracing back centuries.

So long as the pores of the shell can be sealed to prevent the exchange of air and its penetration into the egg contents, then freshness can easily be maintained for quite extended periods. In these matters Asia, and China in particular, have a particularly successful and interesting record that has lasted to the present day. Notable examples are:

Century Eggs (in Chinese: pinyin), also known as preserved egg, hundred-year egg, thousand-year egg and millennium egg, is a Chinese cuisine ingredient made by preserving duck, chicken or quail eggs in a mixture of clay, ash, salt, lime and rice hulls for several weeks or months, depending upon the method of processing. Sealing the pores of the shell by this mixture or even purely using an alkaline

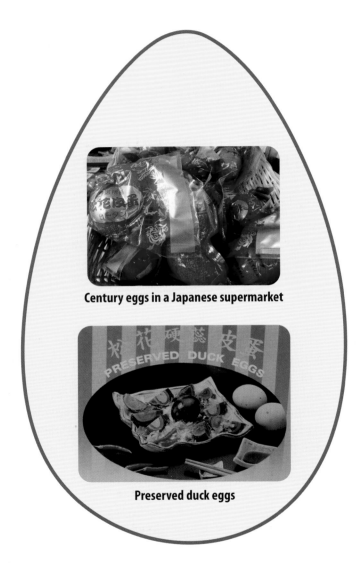

Century eggs in a Japanese supermarket

Preserved duck eggs

clay, assured preservation in times of plenty. The process is not without its culinary frailties. The yolk becomes dark green to grey in colour with a creamy consistency giving off a mixed odour of sulphur and ammonia, while the white takes on the consistency of a dark brown jelly with little flavour, all the result of chemical breakdown of the proteins and fats. The method is still widely practised although modern understanding of the chemistry behind the storage process has enabled some simplification of the recipe and the wrapping of the egg in plastic to achieve appropriate ageing.

Balut. This form of egg preservation is a favourite delicacy among Filipinos and other Southeast Asians. Its basis is a fertilised duck egg containing a near fully developed (16-18 days old) embryo. Following boiling and eaten in the shell, its claim to fame is that of being a good aphrodisiac. The shelf life is only a matter of days but the introduction of the refrigerator has enabled this to be extended to more than a week.

The Tea Egg. This is a favourite presentation of the egg for the Chinese and sold to the communities all over the world. It is simply a hardboiled egg that has been stewed in tea of low quality but high in dark brown tannins. A selection of spices are incorporated in the boiling process with the traditional further addition of soy sauce and black tea leaves. Following boiling, the shell is gently cracked and the boiling water is allowed to seep into the egg contents.

Soy Egg. This is an egg cooked in soy sauce with sugar and spices. Although favoured as a snack, it is also regularly used steamed together with century eggs.

Salted Duck Egg. This is a preserved product made by soaking duck eggs in brine or packing them in damp, salted

Bizarre things that people do with eggs

The biggest eggs

The extinct giant elephant bird (Aephornis maximus) laid eggs one foot in length with a liquid capacity of 2.25 gallons, the equivalent of seven ostrich eggs and more than 12,000 humming bird eggs. When early Arabian and Indian explorers started returning from their journeys along the coast of Africa with stories of gigantic birds many times the size of a man, they also brought evidence in the form of huge eggs, up to three feet in circumference. The eggs that the Elephant Bird laid were larger than the largest dinosaur eggs, and, in fact, they were as large as a structurally functional egg could possibly be.

The largest chicken egg

This was recently found in Jiangyou City, China's Sichuan Province. It weighed 235 grams, 87 grams heavier than a Ukrainian egg previously recognized as the largest egg in the world by the Guiness Book of World Records in 2004.

The smallest egg

The smallest known bird's eggs were two vervain hummingbird (Mellisuga minima) eggs, each less than 1 cm long. They weighed 0.365 g. and 0.375 g.

charcoal. This delicacy is very popular in China but also in Southern Asia where they are also sold coated in a thick layer of salted charcoal paste. The eggs are normally boiled or steamed before being peeled and eaten as a condiment. In spite of the name, chicken eggs may also be used but produce a different texture and taste.

Compared to these exotic Eastern formats, those of the West seem quite mundane and simplistic. Based solely on the principle of covering the pores of the egg shell, a variety of sealants have and are still in use, ranging from waxes to vaseline. The favourite by far and introduced in the early part of the last century was sodium silicate, in culinary terms commonly called "water glass", is a white powder, soluble in water and therefore very easy to make up into solution. Full immersion of eggs enables preservation for up to nine months.

The sodium silicate seal can readily be removed by washing the egg with water. The only drawback to the process was that if the egg was to be boiled, one had to remember to puncture the shell to allow for the expansion of enclosed air. In the second world war and following, the use of water glass was widespread and many happy memories remain of being dispatched to the cold of the domestic pantry and immersing the arm into cold gelatinous "goo" to retrieve the egg(s).

The Pickled Egg. A hard-boiled egg with its shell removed and submerged in a solution of salt, vinegar, spices and seasonings of various sorts for weeks/months. Excellent keeping quality and common to Europe in various formats but also elsewhere in the world.

Q & A

Q. What causes double-yolked eggs?

A. A hen will sometimes lay double-yolked eggs when she is beginning to lay eggs (at about 18 or 19 weeks of age) or near the end of her reproductive life due to hormonal changes. When this happens, the shell forms around two yolks instead of one, creating an egg with two yolks. Double-yolked eggs are safe to eat and cook.

Q. How are eggs sized?

A. Eggs are sized by weight. Eggs in the same carton may look like they are different sizes, but their weight will be within a similar range. The following minimum weights are used to classify eggs into different sizes:

- Peewee eggs - less than 42 g
- Small eggs - at least 42 g
- Medium eggs - at least 49 g
- Large eggs - at least 56 g
- Extra large eggs - at least 63 g

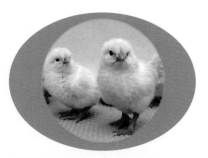

THE WAY FORWARD

All the future exists in the past

It has become clear from the data presented that in nutritional terms the egg has got much for which to be lauded. Concerns and fears on its ability to fulfill a role as a significant and healthy part of our daily diet because of the presence of seemingly "unhealthy" components, most notably cholesterol, and the acceptability or otherwise of production systems potentially leading to dietary contamination, have largely been undermined or entirely eliminated by intensive laboratory and in-field investigations.

Such data would unreservedly suggest that denying or restricting the egg as part of a healthy diet would do more harm than good. However, the matter should not rest solely on the present claims of a healthy credit sheet. From certain sectors doubts will still remain and therefore continuing consideration should be given to assure and even promote further the egg's role in the mainstream of human nutrition.

In the UK and other major European countries the question of housing systems will still remain an issue. Based on sound science, economics and emotion, changes are and will continue to be introduced.

Table 10. Techological ability to enhance food quality

	Egg	Meat	Fish
Vitamin E enrichment	+++	++	+++
Selenium enrichment	+++	+++	+++
Carotenoid enrichment	+++	+	+++

Table 11. Optimal food preparation and serving*

	Egg	Meat	Fish
Boiling vs frying	+++	++	++
Spices and herbs	+++	+++	+++
Serving with vegetables	+++	+++	+++

*under preferential use of olive oil

To this end, new and friendlier housing systems are replacing traditional cages responsible in the past for the major part of egg production. However, in response to public opinion for the need for better quality of eggs produced by healthier and happier hens, free range and free range organic egg production have made significant in-roads into commercial production.

Unfortunately, laudable as the systems might be, the issue is not as simple as supposed. When chickens have access to the outdoor environment, the veterinary control of their health and that of their eggs can become a major issue through transfer of infections from the wild bird population. Although the idea of organic egg production is of good intention, problems arise from the necessity to develop a sustainable model of production.

For example, any idea that the eggs would be free from various pollutants and toxicants such as herbicides, pesticides etc., arising from past or even continuing prodigal usage, is open to severe doubt. The possible prohibition of synthetic vitamins and amino acids in the diet of hens producing organic eggs also requires further thought. In such a situation the amino acid content and composition of the organic eggs would fall far short of that contained in conventional eggs.

Any health threat from the use of synthetic vitamins is very much over emphasised as it has been shown that individual vitamin transfer to the egg is the same whether supplied via feed ingredients or feed supplements. All things being equal, attempts to wholly satisfy the increasing commercial and public demand for organic eggs fails to take into account the limitation of available land to accommodate required production, with the result that the only option would entail reverting back to intensification of some form or other.

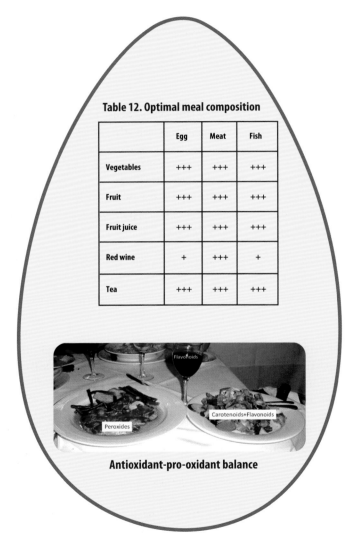

Table 12. Optimal meal composition

	Egg	Meat	Fish
Vegetables	+++	+++	+++
Fruit	+++	+++	+++
Fruit juice	+++	+++	+++
Red wine	+	+++	+
Tea	+++	+++	+++

Flavonoids

Peroxides

Carotenoids+Flavonoids

Antioxidant-pro-oxidant balance

The nutritional benefits to our diet from eggs are clearly of no mean significance. However, with the evidence that the standard egg is readily open to manipulation of nutritional quality, it is seen by many that not only can the egg be cured of any of its "presently seen" nutritional shortcomings but could readily be made the vector for an enhancement in our daily supply of a selection of both major and minor required components.

As mentioned above, in many instances such an enrichment has been little more than returning egg nutritional delivery back to natural values which, in many instances, have been lost due to low price-driven industrial development. The effectiveness of enrichment technology is widely recognised - witness the increasing introduction and acceptance of eggs enhanced with vitamin E, selenium and carotenoids which have elevated the egg into the functional food category.

This potential role for the egg in food production is currently seen as having a particular application to the rapidly expanding attention being given to the anti- and pro-oxidant balances so essential for efficient tissue function and in turn health promotion. The technology to increase the nutritional value of the standard egg in a whole range of directions is being increasingly documented. But questions still remain.

What is the time scale for the egg producers and the retail sectors to move in this direction and, following substantive positive data, see whether it is a technology that finds acceptance by the professionals and consumers alike? Without indulging in any further chemical manipulation, there still remain untapped nutritional roles for the egg in its present form.

Discovery of biologically active compounds are a continuing feature of nutritional science. As has already been pointed out, in nutritional terms the chemical composition of the egg presents a unique storehouse of an exceptional and extensive

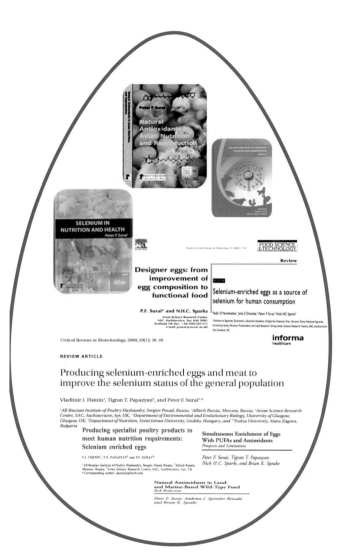

range of essential nutrients, from the macro to micro, with little to show in terms adverse features. This chemical diversity of the egg is such that it is still "open season" for further positive nutritional benefits to be discovered.

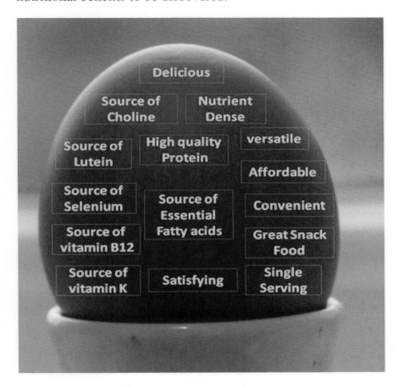

Fifteen reasons to eat eggs

INTERESTING ADDITIONAL READING

1. Surai, P.F. Selenium in Nutrition and Health. Nottingham University Press. Nottingham, UK, 2006, 974 pages.
2. Surai, P.F. Natural Antioxidants in Avian Nutrition and Reproduction. Nottingham University Press. Nottingham, UK, 2006, 615 pages.
3. Fisinin, V.I., Papazyan, T.T. and Surai, P.F. (2009). Producing selenium-enriched eggs and meat to improve the selenium status of the general population. Critical Reviews in Biotechnology 29: 18–28.
4. Fisinin, V.I., Papazyan, T.T. and Surai, P.F. (2008). Producing Specialist poultry products to meet human nutritional requirements: Selenium enriched eggs. World's Poultry Science Journal 64: 85-97.
5. Surai K.P., Surai, P.F., Speake, B.K. and Sparks, N.H.C. (2004). Antioxidant-prooxidant balance in the intestine: Food for thought. 2. Antioxidants. Current Topics in Neutraceutical Research 2: 27-46.
6. Surai, K.P., Surai, P.F., Speake, B.K. and Sparks, N.H.C. (2003). Antioxidant-prooxidant balance in the intestine: Food for thought. 1. Prooxidants. Nutritional Genomics and Functional Foods. 1: 51-70.
7. Blount, J.D., Metcalfe, N.B., Birkhead, T.R. and Surai, P.F. (2003). Carotenoid modulation of immune function and sexual attractiveness in Zebra Finches. Science 300: 125-127.
8. Yaroshenko, F.A., Dvorska, J.E., Surai, P.F. and Sparks, N.H.C. (2003). Selenium-enriched eggs as a source of selenium for human consumption. Applied Biotechnology, Food Science and Policy 1: 13-23.
9. Surai, P.F. and Sparks, N.H.C. (2001) Designer eggs: from improvement of egg composition to functional food. Trends in Food Science and Technology. 12: 7-16.
10. Surai, P.F. (2001). The Super-Egg. Biological Sciences Review 13: 9-12.
11. Surai, P.F., MacPherson, A., Speake, B.K., Sparks, N.H.C. (1999) Designer egg evaluation in a controlled trial. European Journal of Clinical Nutrition 54: 298-305.
12. Leskanich, C.O. and Noble, R.C. (1997). Manipulation of n-3 fatty acid composition of avian eggs and meat. World's Poultry Science Journal 53: 155-183.
13. Noble, R.C. (1998). Manipulation of the Nutritional Value of the Egg. In: Recent Advances in Animal Nutrition, Nottingham University Press, 49-66.
14. Noble, R.C. (1989). Egg lipids. In: Egg Quality; Current Problems and Recent Advances, Butterworth-Heinemann, 159-177.
15. Noble, R.C. and Cocchi, M. (1990). Lipid metabolism and the neonatal chicken. Progress in Lipid Research 29: 107-140.
16. Noble, R.C., Cocchi, M. and Turchetto, E. (1990). Egg fat – a case for concern? World's Poultry Science Journal 46, 109-118.
17. Noble, R.C. (1987). Egg lipids. Poultry Science Symposium 20, 18.
18. Noble, R.C. (1986). Lipid metabolism in the chick embryo. Proceeding of Nutrition Society 45: 17-25.

GLOSSARY

Science uses terminology guaranteed to bemuse and infuriate the non-initiated. The authors have tried hard to pay particular attention to minimising scientific jargon within the text by its avoidance, but if not possible, by explanation in the text: for instance the complexities of the lipid classes and components - see page 56 and following. The following mini glossary is merely a further attempt to lighten any darkness that may still exist. Our apologies if you still remain bemused.

air sac - space at the blunt end of the egg, formed when the inner and outer membranes of the shell separate shortly after the egg is laid.

amino acid(s) - essential nutritional components that sequentially join together to form proteins.

antibody(s)- component(s) released within the body to negate infections.

antioxidant - component that inhibits the oxidative destruction of other molecules.

carbohydrate - major part of the diet to provide energy.

cardiolipin (CL) - important phospholipid of the mitochondrial cell membrane.

carnitine - substance involved in the conversion of fat into energy, also possessing substantial antioxidant properties.

catalase - common antioxidant enzyme for the break up of peroxides into water and oxygen.

chalazae - two spiral bands of tissue within the egg that suspend and hold the yolk centrally within the albumen (white).

chromosome, chromosomal - genetic component of the cell.

chylomicrons - major water soluble particles that enable the transport via the bloodstream of absorbed dietary lipids to locations in the body.

coenzyme - promoter of enzyme function and activity.

coenzyme Q - powerful antioxidant involved in the conversion of dietary components into energy.

denaturation - precipitation/flocculation of proteins.

detoxification - a process of removal or destruction of toxic compounds.

digestion - bodily processing of the diet embracing mechanical and chemical breakdown.

enzymes - protein components essential to chemical reactions within the body.

flavonoids - plant compounds widely distributed in fruit and vegetables.

free radicals - activated molecular oxygen able to damage all biological molecules and responsible for metabolic disorders.

gene expression - ability to develop according to genetic make up.

germinal disc (also called the blastodisc) - small, discrete area on the surface of the egg's yellow yolk and site of the hen's genetic material.

germinal origin - originating from the sexual organs.

gonad - male/female reproductive organs.

glycolipid - molecular carbohydrate/lipid combination.

hormone - specific tissue secretion controlling tissue function and metabolism.

HDL (high density lipoprotein) - group of lipoproteins of specific density range for plasma/tissue exchange of lipids.

immune function - specific role in promotion of tissue protection (immunity).

in situ - "in house" occurrence.

LDL (low density lipoprotein) - group of lipoproteins of specific density range for distribution of dietary lipids, especially associated with cholesterol delivery.

lipid - fat and its many compositional components (see pages 57,61,63, 65,75).

lipoprotein - a solubilised combination of lipids and proteins for plasma delivery.

litter - absorbent material spread on the floor of layer sheds.

macro/micro - large/small.

macula degeneration - reduced visual capacity.

membrane fluidity - physical and chemical state of the cell membrane to allow the free exchange of metabolites.

metabolism - chemical reactions and outcomes within the body.

metalloproteins - proteins in combination with specific metal attachments in order to promote cellular uptake and function.

neonatal - early life.

neurotransmitters - a chemical by which a nerve cell communicates with other nerve cells or tissues e.g. muscle.

Omega 3,6 - simple notation that describes the basic arrangement of the carbon/hydrogen linkages of the two major series of dietary polyunsaturated fatty acids.

ovulation - release of ova from the female gonad.

peroxide/peroxidation - reaction leading to the molecular uptake of oxygen but possessing potential negative effects on metabolism.

prostaglandins - hormone-like compounds associated especially with semen and the prostate gland.

retina - light sensitive membrane at the back of the eye.

RDA/RDI - recommended daily allowance/intake of dietary components (RDA-UK; RDI-USA).

VLDL (very low density lipoprotein) - a group of lipoproteins of specific density range associated with post absorptive nutrients.

Metric Units of Weight.

1 litre (L)	=	1,000 millilitres (ml)
1 ml	=	1,000 microlitres (μl)
1 tonne (t)	=	1,000 kilograms (kg)
1 kg	=	1,000 grams (g)
1 g	=	1,000 milligrams (mg)
1 mg	=	1,000 micrograms (μg)

INDEX

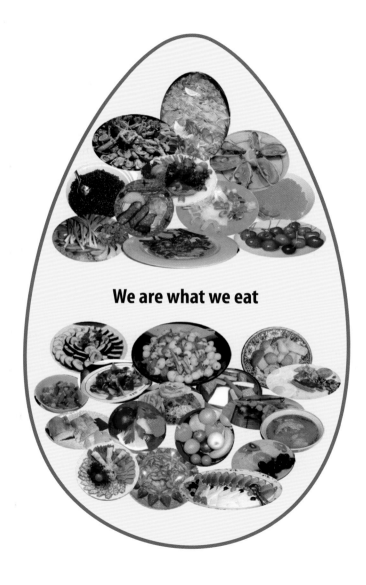

We are what we eat

So, there we are, the end.

The authors would like to think you (the reader) found what we have said is of interest and indeed informative, at least in parts and hopefully *in toto*. Being a couple of academics in science it would have been all too easy to compose something awash with factual detail and terminology and guaranteed to bore the pants off even the most dedicated reader. Scientists tend to be like that. Where we have had to revert to basic science, we would like to think that our efforts to simplify matters are sufficient to overcome any difficulty. We have included much that can be considered as somewhat "off beat" to the subject in hand in the hope that it lightens the load for you.

We clearly leave you to make up your own mind with regard to what the chicken's egg has to offer or can be made to offer. At least the next time you are cracking an egg in the frying pan or impatiently waiting for it to boil, you can muse upon the effort that the humble hen has, day after day, put into what you see before you.

In the case of yours truly, we are now off to try a couple of the best with appropriate trimmings.

Peter Surai and Ray Noble

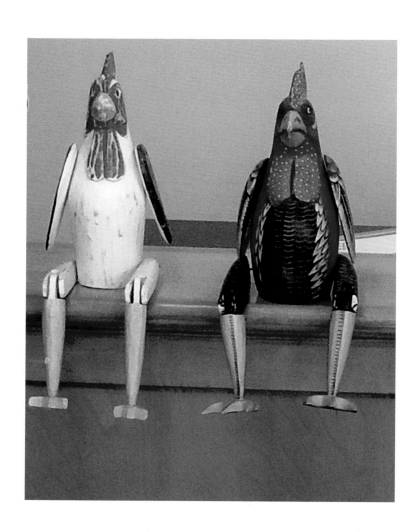